EXPRESSIONS
of an Academic Surgeon

James C. Stanley

to Margie
with great respect
and warm regards!
Peace, Jim
January 2015

EXPRESSIONS of an Academic Surgeon
James C. Stanley

Copyright © 2014
ISBN 978-1-5055-1729-3
Printed by CreateSpace, an Amazon.com Company

CONTENTS

PREFACE

These 20 briefly annotated addresses were selected from more than 450 presentations I've given around the globe during the past four decades as a professor at the University of Michigan. The adage that memory is nonexistent if not written down is certainly applicable to many talks I have listened to in the past. The emotional trail may remain, but the details are gone. My hope is that my words have more value than an isolated academic accolade in a meritocratic arena, and I don't want them to quickly disappear.

Sixteen of these addresses are somewhat personal and philosophic in nature compared to most of my hypothesis-driven talks and peer-reviewed publications that are populated with complicated figures, life-table analyses, and probability statistics. I've also included four formal scientific addresses that are focused on disease entities or interventions that have contributed to the unique reputation of the University of Michigan's vascular surgeons. The latter read like older textbook chapters, but when presented from the podium they represented contemporary ideations.

It is hoped that the thoughts expressed in the following pages might impart a sense of wonder to the reader as to the relevance of science and service in bettering humankind. In the aggregate my words reflect my core beliefs as an academic surgeon. Rereading many of them has awakened me to the diversity and joy of the complex world I've been living in. So be it for others who follow in my footsteps.

MENTORS

Teaching can be extremely dry and often tightly proscribed if limited to the lecture hall. However, the discipline of surgery is still a "hands on" craft and learning how to be a surgeon is not a classroom exercise. In fact it may be one of the few medical specialties that is a holdover from the days of guilds and apprenticeships. What has persisted in the best sense of those days is the value of mentorship. This initial address focuses on my own career and those who helped me. A deep and common thread was woven into my coming of age as a surgeon: the best of my profession distinguish themselves by their mentorship in helping others succeed.

COLLER'S MENTORS AND
AN IGNOBLE ARTERY

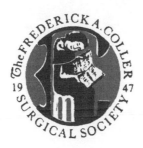

The author was the 36th president of the Frederick A. Coller Surgical Society. This Presidential Address was read before the 41st Annual Meeting of the Society on October 6, 1995, in Bolton Landing, New York.

My comments today are in the form of a very personal statement—not about science, or the terse facts describing the milieu of clinical practice. My comments are meant to reveal a side of me, and perhaps of yourselves, that others rarely see, but perhaps should.

Surgery has evolved by quantum leaps since the days of Fred Coller. The scientific basis for the practice of surgery is exceedingly complex and, combined with the intricacies of dealing with health-care providers and well-intended social planners, often brings chaos to the simplest of our surgical efforts. My method for dealing with chaos, and there seems to be plenty of it, is to frequently reread a copy of a verse written in 1927 by Max Ehrmann, entitled "Desiderata." It bears witness to my chaotic world and perhaps yours. Let me share it with you; you may find some wisdom in its words.

"Go placidly amid the noise and haste,
and remember what peace there may be in silence.
As far as possible, without surrender
be on good terms with all persons.

Speak your truth quietly and clearly;
and listen to others,
even the dull and ignorant;
they too have their story.

Avoid loud and aggressive persons,
they are vexations to the spirit.
If you compare yourself with others,
you may become vain and bitter;
for always there will be greater and lesser persons than yourself.

Enjoy your achievements as well as your plans.

Keep interested in your own career, however humble;
it is a real possession in the changing fortunes of time.
Exercise caution in your affairs;
for the world's full of trickery.

But let this not blind you to what virtue there is;
many persons strive for high ideals;
and everywhere life is full of heroism.

Be yourself.
Especially, do not feign affection.
Neither be cynical about love;
for in the face of all aridity and disenchantment
it is as perennial as the grass.

Take kindly the counsel of the years
gracefully surrendering the things of youth.

Nurture strength of spirit to shield you in sudden misfortune.
But do not distress yourself with imaginings.

So many fears are born of fatigue and loneliness.
Beyond a wholesome discipline,
be gentle with yourself.

You are a child of the universe,
no less than the trees and the stars;
you have a right to be here.

And whether or not it is clear to you,
no doubt the universe is unfolding as it should.
Therefore be at peace with God,
Whatever you conceive him to be.

Whatever your labors and aspirations
in the noisy confusion of life, keep peace in your soul.

With all its sham, drudgery and broken dreams,
it is still a beautiful world.
Be cheerful.
Strive to be happy."

Strive to be happy amid the noise and haste: not always an easy task as a successful surgeon. Finding where you as a person fit, and where your profession fits—at times there seems to be precious little room for both. I never met Dr. Coller, but I'm certainly a product of the Coller Society—a society that doesn't lend itself to vexations of the spirit, is encompassed with high ideals, and for me has brought great happiness. My first recognition of your camaraderie came after I presented a paper on the local program of the 1970 Ann Arbor meeting, a quarter of a century ago. As a third-year resident, who only a year earlier had finally mastered the performance of a McVay herniorrhaphy, you can imagine the sense of awe that overcame me when Chet McVay sought me out at a coffee break during the meeting to give me some insight into the anatomy of the foregut circulation, which had been the topic of my presentation.

My own interest in vascular surgery flourished during my next three years of training, under the guidance of superb Coller Society surgeons, all of whom have addressed you from this podium in the office I now. hold. Jerry Turcotte helped me perform my first carotid endarterectomy; Bill Olsen, my first abdominal aortic aneurysmectomy; and Norm Thompson, my first renal revascularization. It's unlikely that these Coller mentors recall these operations, but I certainly do. I was very impressionable at that time, and remain grateful for their having helped me take my first steps as a young surgeon.

It's really hard for me to believe that I'm the president of this Society. I don't feel that senior or that wise, characteristics I've always attributed to my predecessors. However, my perception as a second-generation Coller trainee as to the importance of this Society has been easy for me to understand if for no other reason than one simple fact—"mentorship."

Coller's mentors and the human condition are the topic of my address. They are intricately intertwined. The principal subject of this topic is an ignoble artery, one of which I've come to understand and respect: the renal artery. Nearly a quarter of the world's English literature on the surgical treatment of this vessel has been written by Coller trainees and the progeny they have mentored.

You may ask, "Why call it an 'ignoble artery'?" Ignoble means "of low character." Well it's rather difficult to label the renal artery a "noble" vessel when it carries a good Chardonnay wine to an organ that turns it into pee. Whatever the case, this artery has been central to my own development as a clinician and academician.

Four individuals have left an indelible mark on me as a student of the renal artery, including two senior surgeons: Bill DeWeese and Ralph Stratton, who were there at the beginning of renovascular surgery; and two others: Bill Fry and Cal Ernst, who provided me with more opportunities than anyone could have ever wished. Their impact on my career, gently applied, was immense.

Bill DeWeese was the reason I chose to become a surgeon. If I could ever mold a father figure for the young, the image would be in Bill's persona. I had been accepted into the Internal Medicine residency program at Michigan my senior year in medical school, when, in an attempt to broaden my horizon, I had a clerkship on the then Private Surgery service. I witnessed my first renal revascularization on that service in 1963, watching Bill and Bruce Stewart make a complex operation appear simple. It was my beginning. It was not Dr. DeWeese's

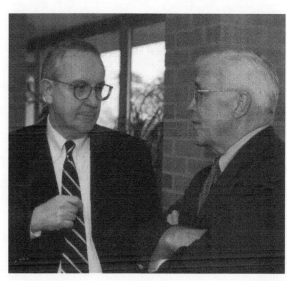

Ralph Straffon and
the author

beginning, as many of you may know. He, in fact, performed the first
aortorenal bypass with saphenous vein. What an accomplishment! Bill's
grace and effervescent mentorship has enhanced many of our lives, and
we and many of our patients are indebted to him.

Ralph Stratton was the second senior surgeon who made a mark
on me. Although I'd heard stories of Ralph's legendary days on the
Michigan gridiron as captain of the football team and as a Urology
resident, my first contact with him occurred at the Coller meeting in
Atlanta over two decades ago. It was there that he spoke with me after
my presentation on the histologic classification of renal artery disease
and shared his insight into the Cleveland Clinic–Mayo Clinic experience on this subject. Ralph may be viewed as someone who mostly deals
with urine, but his contributions to the practice of renovascular surgery were unparalleled. His leadership in this field and impact on his
own trainees, like Andy Novick, reflect the best of mentorship. All the
M-fanfare aside, and even his Presidency of the American College of
Surgeons, the most important thing to me about Ralph were his words
given to me as a young surgeon in 1974.

Bill Fry was the most intuitively correct surgeon in the operating
theater that I've ever known. Bill, by example, taught me how to be a
meticulous technician in performing renal artery reconstructions. He

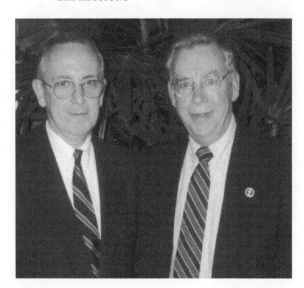

Calvin Ernst and
the author

always encouraged me to be a no-nonsense surgeon and, on many occasions, bailed me out when my grasp not only exceeded my reach, but I
found myself with nothing to hold on to but my other hand. I can still
remember his 1972 home phone number.

Cal Ernst has perhaps been my closest ally around the renal artery.
To a trainee he made the operating room fun. Cal taught me how to
write, which at times was an exasperating but exhilarating experience.
It stuck. If you ever wanted to see academics in the raw, you should have
seen Cal and me go after each other, arguing over each sentence in a
20-page manuscript. You would then understand how professors get
reputations for being weird.

These were the giants in my small world when I was a young surgeon. It was on their shoulders that I stood to gain what I consider a
spectacular view of surgery. How many times have you heard it said
that "I want to give thanks to those upon whose shoulders I've stood"?
It seems to me I've often heard that from someone talking down to me
from a podium, perhaps someone like myself.

But "big deal" for the top of the pyramid idea. The real issue is how
all of us, as surgeons, gain the vision of the few who seem to have rid-
den the shoulders of obvious giants. My answer is, "don't try to find
the giants." There are not as many around as one may think. The crowd

around the people whose shoulders you'd like to stand on is replete with the loud and ambitious, a contentious and unpleasant group at best. We don't often see them at Coller Meetings.

There are better ways for us to succeed in getting the view. Don't ignore the giants but my admonition to you is to nurture the young and let them hold you higher. We can all do this. Mentoring youth well, well enough to carry you up with their energy and creativity, will provide a pretty unique perspective on the human condition. We've done it with our families, our siblings, our children, our friends, and we've certainly done it in the Coller Society. I became a member of the Coller Surgical Society one year after finishing my residency in Ann Arbor. Many recognitions have come my way since, but barring any awards or offices or even the gratitude of some wonderful patients whose renal arteries I've fixed—all of this aside, what has been the most satisfying have been the successes of those I've mentored in the study of the ignoble renal artery. They've provided me with a splendid view of life.

I've mentored 26 junior surgeons on the topic of renovascular hypertension during the past two decades, each of whom has contributed to the literature and my curriculum vitae. Some deserve special mention.

First, Bruce Gewertz was a near brother during his days in Ann Arbor. We did things together that you just wouldn't believe, and we never got caught. Bruce is an exemplary academic surgeon. One of my proudest moments was in hearing him present a classic paper on renal artery dissections at the 1976 Western Surgical Association meeting, a feat easily surpassed by his current role as Chairman of the Department of Surgery at the University of Chicago, one of our country's most prestigious universities. I can't claim credit for Bruce's success, but I can certainly tell you, he's enhanced my vision of our profession.

In a similar vein, Mac Whitehouse's presentation at the Midwestern Vascular Surgical Society meeting in 1980 on the totally occluded renal artery, a series that has not been exceeded numerically in the literature, was one of the first to document improved kidney function by fixing the ignoble renal artery. Mac is as solid as they come. It's difficult for me to convey my satisfaction in having seen Mac succeed as a young academic to his present position, where he leads the surgical services at St. Joseph Mercy Hospital, our sister institution a few miles from the University Hospital.

Vikrom Sottiurai is the third individual who, at times during his training, created an environment where it was difficult to tell who was the mentor and who was the mentee. Vik is a stellar ultrastructural microscopist. His electron microscopy talents in viewing the vasculature are not equaled by any surgeon in our country. Vik presented his work on the ultrastructure of renal artery fibrodysplasia at the International Cardiovascular Society meeting in 1978. This was a classic paper and has not been superseded in the nearly two decades since its publication. To get a better view of an ignoble artery, it would be hard to find someone better than Vik to mentor.

The fourth person is Linda Graham. Her paper on developmental renal artery stenoses presented at the Central Surgical Association in 1979 was the first to document the relevance of multiple renal arteries in central abdominal aortic coarctations. Her letter-perfect presentation brought a deep sense of pride to me. Linda's obviously been a success—a Jobst Award winner, a Coller Council member in our Society, and, a year ago, the first female president of the Society of University Surgeons, previously a bastion of male chauvinism and macho. This was no small accomplishment.

Linda, in particular, has given me a view of our profession that has been difficult to ignore, a view that was recently reinforced by my feelings as to how another woman, Rosalind Franklin, was accepted as a scientist by her peers. As many of you know I've had a deep interest and commitment to the tools of molecular genetics to improve our understanding and treatment of vascular disease. Central to this is an understanding of DNA expression. This summer, while enjoying the pristine landscape of Alaska, I reread *The Double Helix* by Jim Watson, who as you will recall, won the Nobel Prize with Francis Crick for having described the structure of DNA in 1953.

In the last three paragraphs of this classic book, perhaps some of the most important paragraphs in the entire text, Watson made a very strong statement that I can't help but believe he wanted intelligent people to listen to: "Virtually everybody mentioned in this book is alive and intellectually active. All of these people, should they desire, can indicate events and details they remember differently. But there is one unfortunate exception. In 1958, Rosalind Franklin died at the early age of 37."

Rosalind Franklin was a postdoctoral student in Maurice Wilkins's lab when the structure of DNA was being defined. Subsequently, Wilkins shared in the Nobel Prize for describing DNA's structure. Rosalind was important to Watson and Crick's work in retrospect, but when one reads this personal narrative of the discovery of DNA, she was portrayed as an exceedingly difficult person, somewhat angry, and always as a defensive scientist. Sounds a lot like an overworked, underappreciated surgery resident!

Watson then expressed a very personal apology as he continued: "Since my initial impressions of her (both scientific and personal, recorded in the early pages of this book) were often wrong, I want to say something about her achievements." Dr. Watson then describes her later successes as a superb crystallographer, and continues, "because I was then teaching in the states, I didn't see her as often as did Francis (Crick), to whom she frequently came for advice or when she had done something very pretty, to be sure he agreed with her reasoning. By then all traces of our earlier bickering were forgotten and we both came to appreciate greatly her personal honesty and generosity, realizing years too late the struggles the intelligent woman faces to be accepted by a scientific world which often regards women as mere diversions from serious thinking. Rosalind's exemplary courage and integrity were apparent to all when, knowing she was mortally ill, she did not complain but continued working on a high level until a few weeks before her death."

My friends, Jim Watson inscribed these words as a very secure person—a Nobel laureate— and the message is hard to ignore: Don't put aside this half of humankind. They are of great talent and can benefit our scientific profession. To Kathy (a classmate), Jeannie (a fellow resident), Peggy, Maria, Pam, Linda, Usa, Mary, Marian, Elizabeth, and, most recently, Debbie and Rachel: there aren't too many of you. I'm proud you're in the Coller Society. You've brought distinction to our fold; we need more of you.

Lastly, I want to mention three other individuals I've mentored: Jerry Zelenock, Tom Wakefield, and Lou Messina who after eight years on our faculty assumed the Wylie Chair at the University of California, San Francisco, last June, as well as my long-time colleague and teacher, Marty Lindenauer. These four individuals have contributed enormous amounts of energy, time, and ink to the formulation of the Michigan experience with renovascular hypertension. They've been friends who have shored me up when I've needed support, made an often intolerable workload seem light, and have made my being an academic surgeon fun.

Mentorship for me and others who are teachers is easy, but for some of you it may not be so visible. Well, humbug! The contributions that many of you have made to the Coller Surgical Scholarship Fund are a very visible form of mentorship. Believe me; it makes a difference to the young. Just like Chet McVay and Ralph Stratton made a difference to me.

Let me tell you that in my own subspecialty, Milt Bryant has endowed a lectureship in Vascular Surgery that will outlive all of us and will be a major force to encourage the young to reach for greater heights, and become better for it.

Ralph Waldo Emerson said it well, "The best purpose in life is to use it for something that will outlive it." I believe this. I've also benefited from those preceding me who believed it. My strongest sense of indebtedness to all of those who have helped me is to do the same for my own students. We all have opportunities. Take a good look at your own talents and resources. Think of what you can do—and just do it.

Charles Rob, who is considered the father of modern carotid artery surgery, celebrated his 80th birthday in San Francisco a few years ago. On that occasion, a poem by Will Allen Dromgoole was read. It was likely first published in 1900. It's entitled "The Bridge Builder." It has to do with mentorship. I have taken the liberty to slightly alter a few words to reflect both genders representing the youth. You will understand why I'm sharing it with you.

An old man going a lone highway,
Came at the evening, cold and gray,
To a chasm, vast, and deep, and wide.
Through which was flowing a sullen tide.

The old man crossed in the twilight dim;
The sullen stream had no fear for him;
But he turned, when safe on the other side,
And built a bridge to span the tide.

"Old man," said a fellow pilgrim, near,
"You are wasting strength with building here;
Your journey will end with the ending day;
You never again will pass this way;
You've crossed the chasm, deep and wide,
Why build you this bridge at the evening tide?"

The builder lifted his old gray head:
"Good friend, in the path I have come," he said,
"There followeth after me today,
Youth, whose feet must pass this way.

This chasm, that has been naught to me,
To those fair-haired youth may a pitfall be.
They, too, must cross in the twilight dim;

Good friend, I am building this bridge for them."

Most of my professional life has been centered on mentoring and managing the ignoble renal artery. It's been a great adventure. As I've gotten older, things have become more complex, but my perspective is perhaps clearer. Let me tell you, I consider myself a very lucky person. I'm lucky to have had supportive parents; a loving and patient wife, Nancy; great kids, Tim, Jeff, and Sarah; a chance to be a surgery resident at Michigan; an unreal opportunity to be part of a great medical faculty; and lucky to have served as your president.

Whenever I wonder, why the toil, why the extra effort, why the sacrifice? It's rather clear: it's for the fair-headed youth whose feet must come this way. They're the future of our Society. They're the future of our profession. In fact, they're sort of like we were…years ago.

Peace.

LEADERS

There have been many notable leaders in the Surgical Sciences. Some may have been destined for this role since childhood. Others have a slow evolution to leadership over what is often a tortuous road. Drs. Coller, Bryant, and Szilagyi all had different roots and paths. Each had University of Michigan ties to their eventual leadership, which deserve our attention.

2

YESTERYEAR, YESTERDAY:

FREDERICK A. COLLER AND MILTON F. BRYANT

The untimely death of Milton F. Bryant, the 38th Coller Surgical Society president, left a void in the 44th Clinical Meeting of the Society when his presidential address would have occurred. At the request of the Society's Council the following talk was delivered on October 10, 1997, in Osage Beach, Missouri. It was meant to be a solemn fulfillment of what would have been Dr. Bryant's time at the podium.

I wish to speak to you of ourselves and the lives of two of our members: Frederick A. Coller and Milton F. Bryant. Milt Bryant, our President, lost his life in a tragic automobile accident just months ago that robbed him of the opportunity to address us today at this very hour. He had taken voluminous notes on Dr. Coller, had spoken to many of you who preceded him in the office of President, had received from Jean Coller Allen many mementos of her father, and had even visited Marion Jenner, Dr. Coller's OR nurse, to get some inside scoop on the "Boss." Milt seemed to revel in the burden and joy of preparing his presidential address, but fate interceded. His friends and family are greatly diminished by his loss—a loss which is our loss.

Milt revered Frederick A. Coller and the times of yesteryear. Let me remind you that this year is the 110th anniversary of Dr. Coller's birth, and it's been a third of a century since his passing. My sincere desire is to honor Milt's memories of Dr. Coller and our memories of Dr. Bryant, who it seems was here only yesterday. Yesteryear and yesterday of these two individuals hold a very special place for all of us today. A bit of us is probably visible in them, and surely a bit of them is in us.

Dr. Coller's early years were very influential in his later life. He was born in Brooklings, South Dakota, to a Michigan-trained physician and a mother who he said had the "brains" in the family. Fred Coller excelled as a student at South Dakota State College where he received his B.S. in 1906 and M.S. in 1908, before heading to Harvard where he was granted an M.D. degree in 1912. He was not average. He was an outstanding collegiate athlete playing basketball and running the 100 in 10 seconds. He was a serious student in the sciences, especially pharmacy and chemistry, something that served him well at Harvard where he graduated cum laude and was a member of AOA. He was even president of his medical school class.

His success grew during his training years, particularly during his surgical residency at the Massachusetts General Hospital. There he was exposed to the thinking of eminent scholars like Cannon, and surgeons like Cushing and Scudder. Talk about the great!

Dr. Coller was the consummate physician and surgeon. First during a brief stint in private practice in Los Angeles, and then for 37 years from 1920 to 1957 at the University of Michigan, followed by a seven-year conclusion to his professional practice at St. Joseph Mercy Hospital. There is no doubt that the sun rose and set for him at the University of Michigan. There he was indeed the "Boss," someone who trained more than 200 of his kids to become surgeons, who queried the unknown, and who awoke the passion in many who would serve mankind—and who helped many, including Milt Bryant, who was proud to be among the "Coller-Trained."

His leadership became increasingly visible in his military days. As a resident he traveled with the First Harvard Unit to France in 1915 for a brief tour. He returned to Europe after three additional months of residency in Boston, where he was the Assistant Chief of the American Women's Hospital in England. This was followed by his re-entry into the Army after he finished his training and had entered practice in Los Angeles. This third trip to Europe was with the 91st Division from 1918 to 1919. He was a dashing military figure, and many years later left the service of his country as a lieutenant colonel.

Perhaps the most important event during his military years was his marriage at Camp Lewis in 1917 to a Michigan-bred girl and Vassar woman, Jessie Edwards Bernsen, who many of you knew so well. With

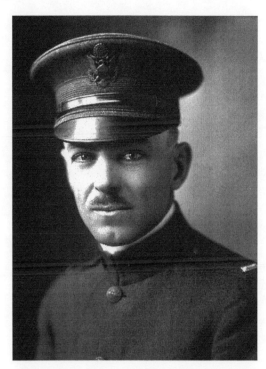

Captain Frederick Coller
in the Army, c. 1918

Fred she raised their two daughters, Carolyn and Jean. Carolyn passed away but our Society has been very fortunate to have Jean attend many of our meetings, including today's gathering.

Milton F. Bryant's early days were very different than Dr. Coller's. He was born in Blakely, Georgia, so called Early County, a small town located in South Georgia. He was raised in a very poor family that had lost their farm in the Great Depression, and like many others he lived in a home without running water or electricity. His mother was the breadwinner. His father was quite infirmed with near deafness and near blindness. His mother persevered and like Dr. Coller's mother made no small bones about the importance of education. That conviction and support saw Milt thrive at school.

He graduated from Blakely High School in 1942 as the recipient of the Harry Stone Award as the most outstanding male student. He then entered Gordon Military Academy as a Naval Cadet in the V-12 program, a program that opened many doors for Milt, allowing him to attend Mercer College where he played both baseball and football. He graduated with a B.S. degree just two years after finishing high school and entered the University of Michigan Medical School the next year, with another young Georgian in the V-12 program—Bill Oliver, who many of you know rose from his roots in Plains, Georgia, to become the Chairman of our Department of Pediatrics.

Following medical school Milt entered the surgical residency at Michigan, where like most of you he learned both the art and science of surgery. He had early leanings toward neurosurgery but eventually chose a career in general surgery and exhibited a budding interest in the evolving discipline of vascular surgery.

Milt's military years followed his Coller training when he entered the Army as a Captain. He served first at Fort Collins, and then as Chief of Surgery at the 11th Evacuation Hospital in Japan. If he learned to stand and think at Michigan, he learned to walk and operate in the military.

Milt married Atchie Woodruff during the last year of his residency in surgery, and it was during those Ann Arbor days that they had their first child, Suzanne. Jonathan, and Douglas were born after he returned from the Army and established a practice in Atlanta. He served on the faculty at Emory University, established a Research Laboratory at Piedmont Hospital, and during his private practice endeavors in Atlanta was very productive. He published nearly 70 articles, most of which related to vascular disease.

He loved blue-water sailing, skiing at Vail, and traveling with his family. His children continue to reside in Georgia. Suzanne lives with her children in Jasper; Jon lives with his family in Stateboro, where he is a Professor of History at Georgia Southern University; and Doug lives in the Atlanta area with his family, where he manages one of Georgia's most successful wine and spirit dealerships, first established by Milt. His mother, Beulah, is 95 and lives with his sister in Florida. His brother, Billy, lives in Atlanta; and we all know his sister, Jo Ann, who is married to Bill Crenshaw, one of our members.

Clearly, Milt enjoyed many of the perks of a successful practice, but all was not roses. As many of you know Milt entered the hospital twice for the treatment of severe depression, during the most productive of his professional years. Many of you in this Society helped Milt regain his

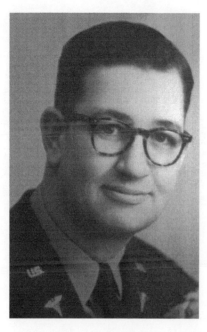

Captain Milton Bryant in the
Army, c. 1952

confidence during these times. Milt deserves great credit—for with the
help of family and friends he came back. After all, it's where you come
out that counts, not where you've been.

So there it is: two men, two eras, two careers—academic and private
practice, two different backgrounds—an affluent physician's son, and a
poor family's son from South Georgia. Apples and oranges perhaps, but
maybe not.

The fact of the matter is that these two men shared many things in
common. Both were considered athletes in their younger years, less
so in their more senior years. Both played golf. Milt shot in the 80's
while he was in his 60's. Both could occasionally be seen at the beach;
Milt, who dressed boldly, probably attracted more attention. Both were
very dapper—Fred Coller could have been in the movies; Milt had his
Ferrari. Both could spend an afternoon at the track. Milt seemed to win.
Both hobnobbed with the famous—Fred Coller with the physiologist
Pavlov in Paris in the 20's; Milt with the entertainer Gene Shalit two
years ago.

Fred Coller and Milt Bryant both loved the glitz of the robes: Dr.

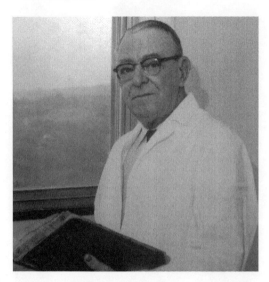

Frederick Coller at the
time of his retirement,
c. 1959

Coller as president of the American College of Surgeons, and as an Honorary Fellow of the Royal College of Surgeons, Edinburgh and England; and Milt as a member of the Camaraderie de Bordeaux. But don't let the robes cover up the people. In fact, they were sort of like the rest of us underneath; Dr. Coller often wore penny loafers, even with his robes. Now that's a classic Ann Arbor town man.

Both liked a good drink and good party—Dr. Coller liked bourbon; Milt liked wine. Remember the Atlanta Coller Meeting and our formal dinner with the Duchin Band; that was vintage Bryant. The real difference in their involvement with the 2-chain-hydrocarbons was that Milt made it a business. He introduced fine wines to Georgia. Today under his son Doug's leadership his spirit stores are among the top three in the state with 12-plus-million dollars in sales each year. Both liked to smoke—Dr. Coller, his cigarettes and pipe; Milt, his cigars. But again, Milt made this a business, retailing thousands of dollars of stogies from his shop's walk-in humidors each year.

In their later years both seemed most at home with the children. Clearly, it was a delight for Milt to see the eyes sparkle in the uncluttered mind of his grandchildren. These were special times for both men.

Dr. Coller's later years were somewhat bittersweet. He did not wish to retire, but he did. He retired as the most distinguished surgeon the University of Michigan has had—and will probably ever have. He left a

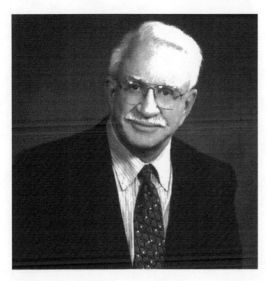

Milton Bryant, 1995

legacy of excellence, of developing fertile fields for inquisitive minds, of healing broken bodies, and a legacy of the Coller Society founded by his trainees.

Dr. Bryant regrouped in his retirement. He returned to his first love, Margaret Boyett Arnold, who was a grade school and high school sweetheart and who was class valedictorian at Blakely High School. She clearly brought great happiness to Milt in recent years. They attended recent Coller Meetings together and traveled the world with each other. But for a split second on a highway, Milt would be here today and Margaret would be at his side. But Margaret has done something very generous to honor Milt, the University of Michigan, and the Coller Society. She has endowed the Milton F. Bryant–Margaret Boyett Arnold Award which will allow a young University of Michigan student, resident, or fellow to attend our annual meeting, as long as we shall be. That is very special.

Milt had some dreams—and some came true. Five years ago he endowed a University Lectureship in his name, something that has deeply enriched the University of Michigan community. Many of you will recognize the names of the lecturers: Mac Perry, a superb vascular surgeon, who in addition attended John Kennedy's last hour in a Dallas operating room on that fateful day in 1963; Jessie Thompson, the father of carotid endarterectomy in our country; Christopher Zarins at Stanford, a member of our Society. Sir Norman Browse, who has headed up

England's Royal College of Surgeons and has been Chief of St. Thomas' in London, will be the Bryant Lecturer next spring. Dr. Bryant was proud of this Lectureship, and there is no doubt that Dr. Coller would have been proud of Milt for having returned to Michigan a little of what it had given him.

So that's it. Dr. Coller, and what was yesteryear; and Dr. Bryant, and what seems to have been yesterday. But you know we all must live today; none of us know if we will have a tomorrow. My friends, there must be some part of us in these two men that holds a message for us today. It should not be so hard to see: do good works and share your love. That's what Fred Coller and Milt Bryant were all about. It's what we should be about.

Peace.

3

D. EMERICK SZILAGYI:
THE STUDENT, SURGEON, SCIENTIST,
AND CONSCIENCE OF VASCULAR SURGERY

This work was read on December 8, 1994, in honor of D. Emerick Szilagyi, as part of a Northwestern University Symposium held in Chicago, Illinois. It was subsequently published in expanded form as a chapter in Advances in the Treatment of Ischemic Extremities, JST Yao and WH Pearce, editors, 1–10, Norwalk, Connecticut: Appleton & Lange, 1995.

D. Emerick Szilagyi is one of a small number of courageous and innovative physicians who established the foundation for the operative treatment of vascular diseases. This brief biographical sketch of his life as a student, surgeon, scientist, and conscience of vascular surgery is offered as a measure of respect to him as he sits with us today.

The Student

Dr. Szilagyi's early education took place in Hungary. He was born in Nagykároly in 1910. Emerick was rambunctious as a young child and was intellectually precocious. His education as a youth occurred in Kolozsvár, a community that he considers his hometown. His was a classical education in the true sense of the Austrian system, involving rigorous academic discipline. He was strikingly handsome as a late teenager when graduating from the gymnasium.

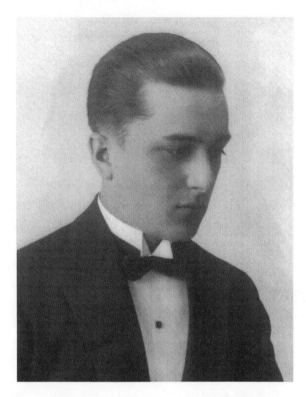

D. Emerick Szilagyi at the time of completing his studies at the gymnasium in Kolozsvár

Dr. Szilagyi subsequently enrolled as a student in the medical sciences at the University of Kolozsvár. He transferred six months later to the Sorbonne in Paris, where he attended science classes of more than 600 students. Each student wore a white coat with an identifying number so that he might be queried by the instructor. This was a demeaning experience to Emerick. Given his strong-willed personality, Dr. Szilagyi elected to return to Hungary, where he then attended the University of Debrecen as a medical student. After being there for two years, in the late spring of 1931, he and his brother traveled to the United States, crossing the Atlantic aboard the *Leviathan*. His father had died when Emerick was a child and his mother remarried and had moved to Detroit with his new stepfather.

His mother had persuaded them to undertake this trip under the guise that it would be a visit for a few months. Once in the United States, she convinced Emerick and his brother to stay. Great unrest existed within European communities as Hitler was rising to power. The concern that their homeland might become the pawn in yet another world war underlay much of her concern. Her intuition proved correct.

As a new arrival in the United States and with citizenship already derived from his mother's having become a citizen earlier, Emerick set about to continue his education. At the University of Michigan, Dr. Szilagyi pleaded his case to Frederick G. Novy, a world-renowned bacteriologist. Dr. Novy had been portrayed as a brilliant scientist in the novel Arrowsmith, written by Sinclair Lewis, who resided in Ann Arbor.

Dr. Novy was a rather imposing individual in the University's medical community. Although Dr. Szilagyi had a near-perfect academic record in Europe, he had not completed the prerequisite English course for admission to medical school. In recognition of his determination, Emerick was asked by Dr. Novy to enroll in the literary school, where he could complete the required course in English. At the same time, he was permitted to take anatomy, physiology, biochemistry, and bacteriology with the entering freshman medical school class. Emerick received an A in English and, having passed muster for Dr. Novy, he began his second year in Ann Arbor as a full-fledged sophomore medical student.

The Surgeon

Upon completing medical school in July 1935, Dr. Szilagyi was accepted into the University of Michigan's Surgical Training Program. He spent the next year as an intern at no pay, other than food and uniforms, rotating through the various medical specialties at the University Hospital. He spent his second year as a senior intern rotating through all the surgical disciplines of the day, at a salary of $20 a month. Dr. Szilagyi then accepted an appointment as a teaching assistant in the Department of Pathology, working for the chairman, Carl Weller, a distinguished anatomic pathologist. He continued in this role for the next two years, from 1937 to 1939.

Following his days in the Pathology Department in Ann Arbor, he applied for and was accepted as an assistant resident in surgery at Henry Ford Hospital. Acute illnesses were more commonplace and nearly all the patients were private, representing the elite of Detroit society and its suburbs. A strong academic atmosphere had been established there by the Chairman of the Surgical Services, Roy D. McClure. He was a Johns Hopkins -trained surgeon and one of Halsted's famous "chosen 17." It was a great fit for Emerick.

At completion of his surgical residency in 1942, he took a two-week vacation with the intent of reporting to active duty in the armed forces. However, Dr. McClure requested that he consider replacing Dr. Kenneth Waddell as Medical Director of the Ford Rubber Plantation in the Amazon valley of Brazil. At the time, Emerick's brother was serving in the armed forces in the South Pacific. It is of historical note that he had no visa when the time carne for his departure to Brazil. A young statesman by the name of Nelson A. Rockefeller working at the InterAmerican Affairs Office interceded with a telegram that allowed Emerick to leave the United States for the Amazon.

When Dr. Szilagyi arrived at the plantation, he was assisted by three Brazilian doctors, whom he supervised. He learned Portuguese quickly and well. Emerick performed nearly 600 operations during his two and a half year sojourn in Brazil, in a small hospital with one operating room and nearly 70 beds. The procedures were undertaken daily from 6 a.m. to 11 a.m., when it became so hot that further work proved impossible. As Emerick noted, he operated on all the organs except the brain and heart.

His surgical adventures in the jungle were clearly a competence and confidence builder, unlike what many young surgeons of the day might ever have experienced. He developed such respect for being versatile that he rejected the establishment's traditional wisdom that a surgeon should do only what he had been trained to do. This was an irrational thought that his experience refuted.

In 1945 Dr. Szilagyi returned from Brazil to Henry Ford Hospital, where he was appointed Assistant Surgeon and for one year served as the chief surgical resident. Shortly thereafter, he organized the second of two surgical divisions within the Department of General Surgery. He served as chief of this division until 1966, when he became Chairman of Henry Ford Hospital's Department of Surgery.

Dr. Szilagyi's first vascular operation, other than a simple embolectomy, was performed in 1951 and consisted of a superficial femoral artery endarterectomy for a segmental occlusive lesion. Emerick maintained an extensive vascular surgical practice until his retirement from the operating theatre in 1984.

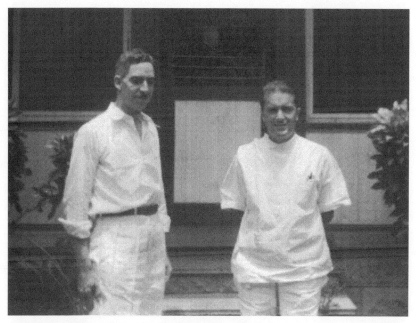

Dr Szilagyi and a colleague at the Plantation Clinic

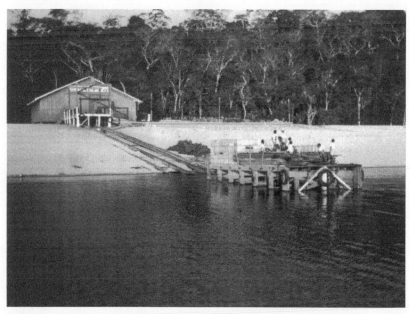

The entrance to the Ford Rubber Plantation in Brazil's Amazon Valley

The Scientist

Few vascular surgeons have made as many notable contributions to their profession as has Emerick Szilagyi. Perhaps his most lasting impact related to his very precise and complete documentation of outcomes following reconstructive arterial surgery. Although he was one of the leading pioneers in the performance of aortic surgery in the 1950s, it was his follow-up of these procedures that awakened the scientific community. His studies on the natural history of aortic aneurysms and their surgical treatment represent classics, as do his clinical publications on reconstructions of aortoiliac occlusive disease and femoropopliteal occlusive disease. Many of his contributions brought a sobering realism to our understanding of vascular surgery.

D. Emerick Szilagyi is best known for his application of statistics to clinical outcome studies. This lent lasting credibility to his work. Prior to Dr. Szilagyi's setting this standard, results were often simply labeled "early" or "late." The fact is that the Henry Ford Hospital Vascular Registry was the first comprehensive compilation of outcome data for vascular surgery patients in the United States. This effort, conceived and initiated by Emerick in 1956, clearly preceded computerized databases familiar to today's practices, and epitomized his understanding of what it meant to be a scientific clinician.

The Conscience

For more than half of his life, D. Emerick Szilagyi has been a familiar and resolute fixture at surgical meetings. Invariably, he sits in the front of the hall near the speaker's lectern and is a visible symbol of integrity in science. There is little question that Emerick's thoughts were molded in part by his indirect lineage to William S. Halsted, whom he described as a surgeon whose "outlook was uncompromisingly altruistic and honest" and whose approach was "consistently original and rigorously scientific." Vintage Halsted. Vintage Szilagyi.

In describing a physician's enigmatic image, Emerick notes: "Born of sick man's primitive instinct of self-preservation, the image of the physician as a man of learning, of superior moral obligations, and of devoted willingness to serve has brought forth a relationship between physician and patient that best fulfills the patient's needs and best rewards the physician." Emerick believed that a physician must sustain that image. He stated: "He must live by the commandments of the method of a scientist, by the rules of a seeker of truth, while nurturing the gentle art of humanistic medicine and while rejecting the allure of the false world of mechanistic, regimented science. He must carry the burden of the ethical-moral dictates of his tradition while the appeal of moral laws in a libertine society around him is growing dimmer."

Perhaps in no other period than when he served as editor of the *Journal of Vascular Surgery* from 1984 to 1990 was his influence on his discipline more resounding. His high standards were reflected in the visible success of this new periodical. He also had some heady advice for those of our profession who may be unknowing recipients of untruthful reports in the literature when he noted that: "The reader of scientific publications has an effective way of reducing or canceling the impact of scientific falsehood. Scientific communication is a give-and-take affair. The listener or reader of these scientific reports, particularly those that claim to represent new and important information, should consider them with friendly but abiding skepticism and accept the conclusions after a leisurely interval of watchful waiting. Delay in acceptance of a worthy idea only postpones the day of its benefits. Prompt acceptance of a concept that is untrue, harmful, or both, enlarges the damage it may do."

Vascular surgery stands indebted to his wisdom. We need to be responsible to ourselves.

Acknowledgment: Dr. Szilagyi spent many Thursday afternoons of focused conversation with the author about his earlier life and career that made this biographical sketch a reality. Each afternoon I left his office with pages of notes detailing the candor and insight he shared with me. It proved both exhilarating and humbling to be in his presence during those hours. I felt honored that he had taken me into his confidence, and I think my work passed his approval. During my presentation at the Northwestern Symposium in Chicago, I noted tears on his cheeks as he sat silently in the second row of the auditorium. For that I felt he must have believed that I'd served his legacy well.

4

D. EMERICK SZILAGYI:
A PERSONAL REFLECTION

My comments as follows were read at the funeral of Dr. Szilagyi, who died peacefully on November 1, 2009, at the age of 99 years. The memorial service was held on November 6, 2009, in Royal Oak, Michigan.

D Emerick Szilagyi was a singular man, and his messages for many generations of patients and physicians were part and parcel of his singularity: "Don't be among the timid"; "Do it and do it right"; and "Don't delude yourself—be sure what you do is lasting."

He stands among a few courageous individuals who more than a half-century ago established the specialty of Vascular Surgery. In the most resolute manner, Emerick sowed seeds that we should all cultivate in our own lives and our progeny's lives—the things that made him a person of intellect, a man who held others in high expectation, and someone of the highest moral character, someone who was a singular man.

Shortly after arriving in the United States from his native country of Hungary, he pursued his life's desire to enter the field of medicine. His student days at the University of Michigan from 1931 to 1935 were exemplary; he graduated with his medical degree cum laude and a commitment to become a surgeon. During his subsequent residency days at Henry Ford Hospital, he wrote a thesis on surgery in infants, which was the basis for his being awarded a Master of Science degree from the University of Michigan in 1940. He was just 30 years old and less than a third of his life had passed, but he had set high standards for himself and he had succeeded.

Current generations are not likely to know of the impact Emerick

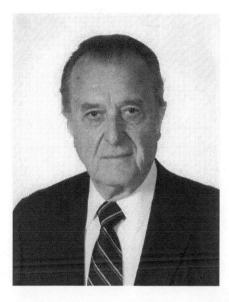

D. Emerick Szilagyi, 1910-2009

had on the practice of surgery. His scientific rigor was the standard followed by the very best of vascular surgeons. To be less was not acceptable. For more than half of his 99 years, Emerick was a familiar and somewhat stoic fixture at surgical meetings. Invariably, he would sit in the front of the hall near the speaker's podium, being a visible symbol of integrity in science. He provided great insight into being a proper surgeon, the best practice of surgery, and the importance of honesty in science. On more than one occasion, if you didn't have significant p values you didn't count. He was the conscience of our specialty and he made a difference.

Emerick once stated his opinion of a surgeon: "He must live by the commandments of the method of a scientist, by the rules of a seeker of truth, while nurturing the gentle art of humanistic medicine and rejecting the allure of the false world of mechanistic, regimented science. He must carry the burden of the ethical-moral dictates of his tradition while the appeal of moral laws in a libertine society around him is growing dimmer." This quote from a presidential address at one of our learned surgical societies more than 40 years ago is vintage Szilagyi: "We need to be responsible to ourselves."

Emerick had a major impact on my own life; it began in earnest when he invited me to be his associate editor of the *Journal of Vascular*

Surgery. That was in 1985, a year after the *Journal* was first published, 24 years ago. He became my mentor, and I was a serious student. I carried reams of notes home after each session of reviewing submitted manuscripts with him, face to face; but most importantly I carried home a deep sense of admiration for him as one who never played favorites or let preconceived thoughts trump newly discovered scientific data. Those are lessons I have never forgotten.

It isn't hard to sum up Emerick's life. He was a voracious reader and clear thinker. As the conscience of the discipline of Vascular Surgery, he had no peer. As a friend and mentor I couldn't have asked for more.

Emerick, I will miss you. Godspeed my friend.

SCIENCE'S SPECTRUM

The underpinning of modern medicine is good science. It is the most important ingredient in the understanding and prevention of disease, and is essential in advancing contemporary care of the ill. Good science is part of a spectrum. My two addresses on this topic are poles apart. The first underscores the need for ongoing assessments of existing clinical practices as a necessary step to ensure quality care. The second, a foray into the basic elements of life itself and the subject of gene therapy, occurred at a time when altering our genetic response to diseases was considered easily achievable. Within the spectrum represented by these two extremes are many bench-to-bedside investigations, of which the author has been a fortunate participant. The most personally rewarding occurred in the Jobst Laboratories where I served as the Director from its inception in 1989 until 2004. A litany of distinguished investigators and projects emerged from these laboratories during the past quarter century.

Many clinician-scientists had roots in the Jobst enterprise, including: Linda Graham MD, Louis Messina MD, Thomas Wakefield MD, Bengt Lindblad MD PhD, Jan Brunkwall MD PhD, Thomas Huber MD PhD, Rajabrata Sarkar MD PhD, Keith Ozaki MD, Peter Henke MD, and Gilbert Upchurch Jr MD. In addition to Drs. Lindblad, Brunkwall, Huber, and Sarkar, whose work in the Jobst Laboratories was the basis for their PhD theses, both David Vinter PhD and Brenda Cho PhD received their doctorates based on experiments performed in our laboratories.

Vascular Surgery and the Jobst Laboratories at the University of Michigan have been a cauldron of good science.

5

BIOMEDICAL SCIENCE AND
VASCULAR SURGERY

The author was a founding member and the 3ʳᵈ president of the Midwestern Vascular Surgery Society. This is his Presidential Address presented at the 4ᵗʰ Annual Meeting of the Society, on September 26, 1980, in Cincinnati, Ohio. An expanded work emanating from this address was published in Surgery 89:705–9, 1981.

I believe it is essential to have a more robust coupling of biomedical science with vascular surgery. Unfortunately, the increasing rate of introducing new technology does not ensure better care. In fact, there has been little improvement the past five to 10 years in outcomes following many common reconstructive vascular procedures—doing more, but not necessarily better. As a group who, more often than not, deal with palliation, I would submit to you that "more and not better" is an unacceptable tenet for us to repeat after one another, year after year. A need for better science is a fitting topic for the Midwestern Vascular Surgical Society, whose identity is closely tied to Charles C. Guthrie, MD, PhD, who was a demanding scientist.

From my perspective it seems that the regularity with which relevant clinical advances have occurred in the practice of vascular surgery has been much less during the 1970's, in contrast to the 1950's and 60's, when many contributions to our understanding and caring for patients with vascular disease were truly phenomenal. Development of synthetic materials as arterial substitutes, the use of balloon catheters for arterial embolectomy, and the undertaking of extra-anatomic bypasses, represented tremendous strides in our clinical capabilities. Recently things have been different.

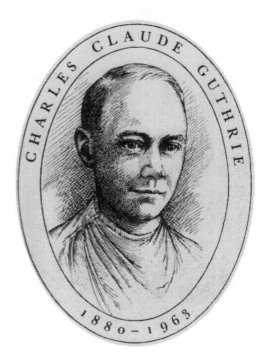

Charles C Guthrie as
depicted on the MVSS
membership certificate

With the exception of noninvasive vascular testing, the past decade has been encumbered with greater concerns regarding the appropriate application of existing knowledge. Who should perform vascular surgery? How should these individuals be trained? What is the minimum operating experience necessary to maintain adequate skills in arterial surgery? Should the occasional vascular surgeon be allowed privileges to perform complex elective reconstructions? Sound familiar? Such moral, economic, and political questions are time-consuming. All of us have been exposed to them, if not at the national level, certainly in our own hospitals. A dominant portion of the energies of many senior vascular surgeons have been directed during the past decade to these issues. Biomedical science has been in second place.

It is conceivable to me that many of the aforementioned diversions have dampened the inquisitive, adventurous scientific spirit so characteristic of our discipline in its earlier days. If I am right, it may be a sad day for all of us. I honestly believe that important advances in our profession will come about more regularly if we demand and support science in the broadest terms. This is certainly as important as our developing means to regulate our practice. Penetrating scholarship, critical attitudes, and the scientific theory necessary for intellectual development and growth are essential ingredients to progress. These things are not a given. They are learned, and we have an obligation to insure their survival. At issue is research.

Research is the action arm of biomedical science and by my standards is easily divided into two types: good research and bad research. It is perhaps by these categories rather than clinical, applied clinical, basic, and a variety of other labels, that most investigative activities should be judged. Certainly when discussing biomedical science related to the clinical discipline of vascular surgery this would seem to be the case.

Many creative contributions have evolved from the most unstructured, least experimentally oriented efforts. Similarly, some of our most profound insights into diseases of the arterial wall, on a cellular and molecular level, represent the culmination of carefully designed laboratory research performed by deft investigators. The fact is that retrospective reviews, prospective clinical research, and vigorous bench investigations all have value to us as clinical vascular surgeons. We should be accepting of any type of research, when the product is good, and be critical of research when it is bad, not when the arena in which it is conducted is out of step with our prejudices.

I would maintain that the vascular surgeon has a unique role in establishing the expectations and direction of many research efforts dedicated to vascular disease. From a practical perspective very few surgical disciplines are as autonomous as vascular surgery. Think about it. We are amongst a distinct minority of surgeons who find themselves primarily responsible for understanding the natural history of a disease, documenting its presence with a variety of our own diagnostic tools, treating patients both operatively and medically, and assuming their long-term care. Unlike the cardiac surgeon who has cardiologists to refer and help care for patients we have few brethren in the clinical sphere to work with, other than ourselves. There are, of course, notable exceptions such as the European angiologists, and outstanding Vascular Internists found at some of our larger institutions such as the Cleveland Clinic and the Mayo Clinic here in the Midwest.

If we are in such a unique position with such broad practice opportunities, then it would seem very important that we accept our unique responsibility to be more than technicians in caring for patients with vascular disease. We must influence biomedical science regarding our discipline. If we don't, no one else will.

Why be concerned? Well, first, much of our understanding of the natural history of vascular disease evolved from longitudinal studies performed in the 1930's, 40's, and 50's that are irrelevant today. Estes's documentation of aortic aneurysm rupture rates and Boyd's documentation of occlusive disease and claudication may represent classic works, but in no way would they pass scientific scrutiny today. It is almost like an awakening to be exposed to a well-documented contemporary investigation that causes us to reassess our earlier convictions concerning a disease process, or even more importantly the appropriateness of some of our most sacred operations. Perhaps we have been too accepting of our heritage.

A second reason to be concerned relates to the tremendous volume of worthless data being generated by well-intentioned writers and published in the contemporary literature. It is almost overwhelming. During the past decade the number of articles relating to vascular disease in the most commonly read American surgical journals has more than doubled.

Although in some sense this may be viewed as laudatory, the vast majority of these contributions represent uncontrolled clinical studies or anecdotal reports with premature claims as to their importance. The basis for what is often misinformation is difficult to clearly delineate. Perhaps it is because there are a limited number of recognized vascular surgeons on editorial boards of many peer-review journals, to protect our interests. Perhaps we as readers have been too accepting of information presented in the literature, being too eager to witness hoped-for advances as occurred frequently 10 to 20 years ago.

This criticism is not meant to sound like an undirected diatribe. Instead, it is addressed to the practical issue of how we practice clinical vascular surgery. The publication quagmire finds me as a teacher often telling students "I don't know." This has not stopped me from saying "I can do." It just means that my judgments of many clinical problems have been served very poorly by the literature. Many elegantly constructed reports present almost incontestable evidence regarding a disease or its treatment exactly the opposite of other equally convincing papers. Let me discuss some particulars.

How does one treat the asymptomatic carotid bruit? Perhaps a better question would be: what is an asymptomatic bruit? Is it auscultated by a physician, noted on the chart, and then discovered during a retrospective review, or does it represent a nontransmitted mid- or upper-cervical neck bruit documented by ultrasonography or phonoangiography? Answering this question by reviewing publications by many vascular surgeons is, to put if graciously, very disquieting. There is ample evidence to suggest that certain asymptomatic bruits may be warning signals of potential neurologic catastrophes. However, no randomized prospective clinical studies of the general population exist to adequately define in a scientifically acceptable manner the natural history of a carotid bruit. Extracranial cerebrovascular arteriosclerosis is a major disease, a common disease, and one we treat all the time. It is simply unreasonable for those of us in a close geographic proximity to have such different perceptions of its meaning, such that many of us regularly pursue invasive studies and operation immediately for asymptomatic bruit associated with carotid disease, while others believe that these bruits should be followed conservatively. Where has biomedical science been in this matter? Where have we been?

Just as ubiquitous as the asymptomatic bruit is the ever changing role of noninvasive studies in evaluating significant extracranial carotid artery disease. Unless we are willing to say that the technician or physician interpreting the results is the critical variable in many of these studies, it seems reasonable to conclude that interests, almost of a proprietary nature, have caused certain individuals to expound the virtues of one testing method over another. Among all topics related to vascular disease the past five years, the noninvasive approach to cerebrovascular disease has been one of the least understood. In Dr. Jack Wylie's recent presidential address before the Society for Vascular Surgery he condemned our collective mentality in pursuing noninvasive studies without critically recognizing their limitations. His remarks may have seemed inappropriate to some of you but they should not be overlooked or ignored. Measurements, as we have repeatedly been reminded by Dr. John Bergan, my immediate predecessor in this office, are essential to the practice of vascular surgery. I believe this firmly. But don't be misled:

mere acquisition of a number on a piece of paper does not guarantee the scientific practice of vascular surgery.

Another dispute relates to arterial reconstructions for lower extremity ischemia in patients with disabling claudication, rest pain, or actual tissue loss. An example is the ominous prognosis of diabetes and heart disease in patients undergoing femoropopliteal bypass, with no survivors noted beyond five years in one widely quoted work. Many other works, including one by our first president, Dr. Szilagyi, have noted very few differences in survival or patency rates of femoropopliteal and distal bypasses among patients with and without diabetes. Now, how do you advise patients with diabetes and a history of coronary disease as to the clinical importance of their illness or durability of potential reconstructive surgery when such disparate data exists in the literature? Where is the science to come from to settle these issues?

If you accept the unsettled nature of selecting patients for extremity revascularization, then the unscientific basis for choosing a specific type reconstruction should be readily understood. The indications for, and results of, profundoplasty or sequential bypasses have yet to be the subject of a well-designed prospective randomized study. Perhaps most disconcerting of all issues relating to femoropopliteal and distal bypass surgery are the solicitous claims of success using various prostheses, especially PTFE. If surgeons reporting good results with PTFE are actually operating on the type of patients they claim, and there is no reason to suspect otherwise, then their techniques must be unlike that of many others who have been unable to achieve similar good results. The reported differences with this graft material are incomprehensible. Would not reasonable randomized studies have contributed more to our assessment of this graft than the polarized clinical experiences currently existing in the literature?

The list of "why be concerned?" subjects is long. As examples, we sorely need accurate answers about: the seriousness of combined coronary artery and peripheral vascular disease; fibrinolytic therapy for venous thrombosis; the efficacy of newer biologic as well as prosthetic graft materials; and certainly the role of percutaneous transluminal angioplasty as an adjunct to, or substitute for, reconstructive arterial surgery. None of these questions will be answered by casual clinical reports, no matter how well intended they may seem, or how elegantly they are written.

If answers to many of these issues are not in, then how can one make rational decisions regarding many common diseases that we are required to treat? The answer is we can't. We can only make expeditious choices, based on our own biases. That is easy. Because of our unique isolation as a discipline, which does everything from diagnosis to treatment to burial, there is no one around to question our actions. Although choices come easy to us as "cutting surgeons," they are not always the correct ones. Need I remind you of sympathectomy for treating hypertension, or even venous disease in the distant past, or the enthusiasm more recently for bovine heterografts? Decisions based continually on our own biases are unacceptable, especially if reasonable biomedical research would afford a more rational clinical practice.

Having expressed considerable displeasure with what I consider an exceedingly important matter relating to our discipline, what would I recommend in the way of solutions?

First, it is my personal conviction that the time to establish a vascular surgeon's critical sense of thinking and judgment related to new knowledge is during that individual's training. Most fellowships are highly geared toward the education of practicing vascular surgery. This is clearly appropriate. The RRC criteria for establishing training programs include no comment concerning primary investigative activities.

It would be my recommendation that regional societies, such as ours, should encourage certain of our young trainees to develop themselves as thinkers as well as doers. In this regard I would submit to you that we establish a Charles C. Guthrie Award for Outstanding Research in Vascular Surgery by a resident or fellow. After all, Guthrie's image is on our membership certificate and he was a stellar scientist. This award should be granted at our annual scientific meeting in association with the presentation of a paper related to biomedical science. There would no restrictions as to whether this work represented clinical or laboratory research. It would simply have to represent the best of good research. Recognition of our young successors, who make outstanding contributions to our understanding of vascular disease, would seem appropriate if we are to insure the truth of our membership certificate legend, which states that the Midwestern Vascular Surgical Society was "founded to advance the science, art and high standards of practice in peripheral vascular surgery." It's of note that "science" is listed first.

Second, it seems that many discrepancies in earlier clinical reports relate to an inadequate definition of the disease process being treated. It would seem that the time is right to develop standard definitions of peripheral vascular disease, in the classic sense. Today it is certainly possible to develop a classification that would define (1) the pathologic lesion, (2) the morphologic character of the lesion, (3) the anatomic extent of the disease, and (4) the functional impact of the disease. Such a simple set of standards would allow us to stage patients, before instituting therapy and judging results. There are precedents to help us, such as the New York Heart Association categories used in assessing cardiac disease, or for that matter the International Coding of Neoplastic Diseases. I would propose that our Society establish an ad hoc committee to study the feasibility of such an effort, with the intent of approaching the national vascular societies or the American Heart Association with such a project.

A third suggestion relates to support, and if you will, a demand for good clinical studies. Robert Condon in his presidential address before the Central Surgical Association was very clear in defining whose responsibility prospective clinical research was. It's ours. Not mine as a university professor, but ours as practitioners. To proceed in practice with an unwillingness to participate in clinical research is like telling our profession to sail in an uncharted sea. It is not only unwise; it is foolish. As next year's immediate past president, and as a holdover on your Council, I will take the opportunity to submit to you two proposals relating to prospective clinical research that this membership can contribute to. Areas of investigation I have in mind involve carotid artery disease, and the use of prosthetic or biologic grafts in lower extremity arterial reconstructions. There is no lack of talent in either the academic or private practice sectors of this Society and your input, individually or collectively, will be solicited.

Finally, I wish to extend my very sincere appreciation for having had the opportunity to serve you as the 3rd President of the Midwestern Vascular Surgical Society. The greatest honor accorded me in this office has been the opportunity to have developed close personal and professional associations with many of you, something that will not be lost as the Presidential office is passed on to my successors.

———————

Context: At the time of this Presidential Address many technologic advances in open vascular surgery were being offered to practitioners with little hard data to justify their use. It was estimated that nearly a fifth of newer arterial reconstructions were often applied in the clinical setting before their benefits had been established. This caused a modest amount of angst among the profession's leaders, including the author.

In regard to the three action items alluded to in the address: The stratifications of many disease states being treated were defined years later by the Society for Vascular Surgery and the two intended prospective clinical studies became part of NIH-initiated and commercial studies.

The Guthrie Award has remained within the purview of the Midwestern Vascular Surgical Society for more than three decades. Charles G. Guthrie held both MD and PhD degrees. Most importantly he was a scientist of great renown and worked hand in hand with Alexis Carrel, where they performed benchmark vascular experiments at his laboratory in Chicago, some of which carried Carrel to the 1912 Nobel Prize in Medicine. Many distinguished clinicians and scientists have received the Society's Guthrie Award since its inception in 1981.

6

MOLECULAR GENETICS,
GENE THERAPY, AND VASCULAR DISEASE

This lecture was presented as an invited address before the 23th Annual Meeting of the Japanese Society for Cardiovascular Surgery on March 5, 1993, in Fukuoka, Japan. At that time there was an extraordinary effort in the United States at bringing gene therapy into the clinical arena. Considerable activity in this field surrounding the vasculature occurred at the University of Michigan in the laboratories of Elizabeth and Gary Nabel, James Wilson, Louis Messina, and the author. Landmark papers emanating from this group were widely published in highly respected journals, including Science 244:1342–44, 1989, and Proc Natl Acad Sci USA 89:12018–22, 1992.

Few areas of research in recent times have generated as much interest among the scientific medical community as has recombinant DNA technology. The ability to define molecular mechanisms that control normal physiologic events or cause pathologic states, as well as the ability to manipulate the genetic control of these phenomena, represent the basis of a broad, new form of medicine. The role of molecular genetics in altering specific disease states within the vessel wall, such as arteriosclerosis and neointimal hyperplasia, is likely to become relevant in the near future.

Molecular Genetics

Double-stranded deoxyribonucleic acid (DNA) constitutes the substance of the 23 chromosomes located in the nucleus of all somatic cells. Four different base **nucleotide molecules** provide the structure of DNA: two purines—adenine (A), and guanine (G); and two pyrimidines—thymine (T) and cytosine (C).

These nucleotides are paired on the two coiled strands of DNA such that an adenine and thymine and a guanine and cytosine are always opposite each other. The couplings of these two nucleotides are known as base pairs (bp). The sequence of the bp defines all encoded genetic information. The usual gene is 2,000 to 3,000 bp in length. There are more than 3 billion bp, or 6 billion of the four individual nucleotide molecules, in the nucleus of each human cell. However, it is estimated that only 15% of these nucleotides have a direct role in the control of cellular activity.

Transcription is the initial process by which genetic information in DNA is expressed in the cell. Under the influence of the enzyme ribonucleic acid polymerase, DNA unwinds preparatory to formation of complementary intermediate **messenger RNA (mRNA)**. This unwinding allows complementary molecules, in a paired fashion, to line up alongside the single strand of unwound DNA. Each nucleotide within the DNA has a pairing with a matching base molecule on the strand of mRNA, except that uracil (U) is substituted for thymine in the mRNA. Further processing of mRNA causes deletion of certain nucleotide segments called **introns** that are believed unimportant. This leaves mRNA segments called **exons** that contain the essential genetic information for protein formation.

Translation is the process by which mRNA initiates protein synthesis. mRNA serves as a template upon which specific amino acids become aligned. These amino acids are part of a three-dimensional structure known as **transfer RNA (tRNA)**. A genetic code exists such that a given three-segment nucleotide sequence on tRNA, called a **codon**, causes alignment on mRNA of one of the 20 amino acids. A total of 64 different arrangements of three-segment nucleotide sequences, (4^3), exist for the 20 amino acids. Thus, some amino acids have more than one codon. The relationship between the codons and amino acids defines the **genetic code**. The amino acids, two at a time, are subsequently merged to form a polypeptide chain. As this process continues, complex proteins are formed within the cell. Because certain amino acids have multiple codons, it should be apparent that the exact gene nucleotide

sequence may be difficult to predict for proteins containing hundreds
of amino acids.

This simplified description of cellular protein production, in reality,
belies a much more complex process. Regulation of gene expression is
under the influence of other nucleotide sequences called **promoters**,
located proximal to the gene on the DNA; and **enhancers**, located at
more remote distances from the gene, both of which bind proteins
that facilitate transcription. Formation of a transcription complex that
positions RNA polymerase at the initiation site of the gene is the result
of multiple DNA-protein and protein-protein interactions.

Recombinant DNA Technology

Recombinant DNA technology involves transfer of foreign DNA into
a different cell's genomic DNA. When a specific gene is inserted into
another cell the cloned gene may be markedly amplified for study, or
used to produce a protein. Essential to this technology has been the
discovery of two important enzymes, **restriction endonucleases** and
ligases, which allow cutting and splicing of nucleotides in a predictable
manner.

Various substances commonly used in clinical practice, such as insu-
lin, growth hormone, erythropoietin, and tissue plasminogen activator
(tPA), are produced by recombinant means. This is made possible by
the transfer of their responsible genes into prokaryotic cells such as
Escherichia coli bacteria, which act as the factory to produce these new
proteins.

Gene transfer may be undertaken in eukaryotic cells and provides
the potential for **human gene therapy**. Gene augmentation may be
achieved by placement of genetic material into the cytoplasmic epi-
somes, a process known as **gene introduction**. It should be noted that
the effectiveness of this type of gene transfer is limited by the cell's lon-
gevity, with cell death terminating any effect of such therapy. A second
method of gene augmentation is by placement of new genetic material
directly into the host chromosome through a process known as **gene
insertion**. This approach allows the therapeutic effect to be passed on
to the progeny of this cell if it divides, and holds a distinct advantage

if stem cells are the recipients of the new genetic material. The current status of gene insertion does not involve specific site-directed insertion.

Genetic material may be introduced into eukaryotic cells by techniques using physical or chemical means, and fusion carriers. Genetic material may also be inserted into eukaryotic cells by the process of transfection, using a number of viral vectors. Included are the transforming DNA viruses, papovavirus and SV-40, as well as certain adenoviruses. The most important development in viral vectors was the identification and use of appropriate murine and avian retroviruses for the transfer of genetic material. These RNA viruses enter the cells, where they reside within the cytoplasm and act as a template for reverse transcription of the genetic information within the virus to form complementary viral DNA. Insertion of a gene of interest into a retroviral carrier provided the basis for gene transfer in many contemporary experiments. A virus must not be able to replicate itself when used for gene therapy. Under most circumstances, there is a deletion of a considerable portion of native viral genome encoding for the proteins necessary for duplication of the virus. This renders the recombinant viral particles replication incompetent.

Integration of the complementary viral DNA strand as a provirus occurs at random sites within the host genome's DNA. Existing technology using viral vectors usually leads to insertion of multiple gene copies into the host's DNA, with their subsequent expression being unregulated. Such unregulated protein production is called **constitutive expression**. Site-specific insertion and **regulated expression** are potentially feasible. The conceptual simplicity of molecular genetics, using recombinant DNA technology as a means of altering a cell's function, makes this form of intervention attractive for application in numerous clinical settings.

Applications of Genetic Engineering to the Vessel Wall

Genetic modification of the endothelium and smooth muscle of arteries and veins has been successfully accomplished by a number of investigators. Certain unique characteristics of endothelium make it an attractive target organ for expression of foreign genes in vivo. Endothelium's immediate interface with the bloodstream allows luminal release of various proteins having a paracrine effect on local surface thrombotic events, or endocrine effects, such as clot lysis and inhibition of platelet aggregation, along the downstream bloodsurface interface. Similarly, because of its close apposition to medial smooth muscle cells, endothelium may influence a number of significant interactions between these two contiguous layers of the vessel wall, especially those involving vasomotion and cellular proliferation.

A number of recent reports relevant to this topic deserve note, including both in vitro and in vivo studies.

Zwiebel and colleagues at the National Institutes of Health (NIH) were among the earliest to document that endothelial cells in vitro could serve as recipients of functioning recombinant genes. Dichek and his colleagues, in a second in vitro study at NIH, transferred the gene encoding for the production of beta-galactosidase and human tPA into cultured sheep endothelial cells. These transduced cells were subsequently seeded onto stainless steel stents of the type applicable for intra-arterial use during angioplasty.

Brothers and his colleagues at the University of Michigan assessed the effect of genetic transduction on canine endothelial cell prostacyclin production and cell growth in vitro. In these studies, canine venous endothelium was transfected with a retrovirus containing the *LacZ* gene responsible for beta-galactosidase production, in combination with the neomycin resistance gene. Transduced cells consistently revealed a slower proliferation rate than normal nontransfected cells in the culture environment.

Nabel and her colleagues at the University of Michigan undertook a series of in vivo studies that documented recombinant gene expression among endothelial cells placed within iliofemoral arteries of Yucatan minipigs after they had been transduced with the *LacZ* and neomycin resistance genes using a retroviral vector. Nabel and her colleagues also documented the presence of in vivo site-specific gene expression following a direct gene transfer without a vector.

In a third in vivo study, Wilson and his colleagues, at the Whitehead Institute and Tufts University, implanted porous Dacron carotid artery interposition grafts in a canine model that had been seeded with genetically modified endothelial cells. The latter were transduced

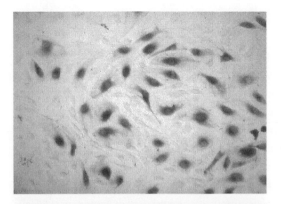

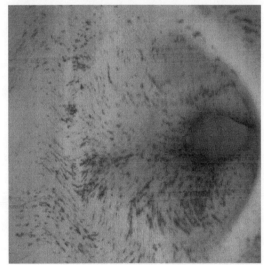

Beta-galactosidase gene expression in retroviral transfected cultivated endothelial cells (upper), and in adenoviral transfected endothelial cells of an intact artery (lower), evident in dark x-gal stained cells

with the *LacZ* gene alone. Grafts examined up to five weeks postimplantation revealed expression of beta-galactosidase activity among the seeded cells and their progeny on the surface of the grafts.

Expression of beta-galactosidase in transduced cells has been used to document the geographic fate of seeded endothelium in lineage studies in our laboratory. Such *LacZ* transfected cells have been seeded on a number of graft substrates, including expanded polytetrafluoroethylene (ePTFE) prostheses placed as thoracoabdominal grafts in dogs. Successful genetic transfer was documented from the progeny of the seeded cells that spread over the graft surfaces during a six-week period of time. Experiments in the author's laboratory, assessing *LacZ* gene expression have been carried out in vitro with both retroviral and adenoviral vectors.

Currently, the use of retroviral vectors limits the size of the gene that may be inserted to approximately 8,000 bp. Similarly, the transfection rate using most retroviral vectors is relatively low and better methods are needed to increase the efficiency of transfection. Furthermore, the constitutive, unregulated expression of protein production by cells that have had random, rather than site-specific, insertion of genetic material into their genome may alter important existing cell functions. Finally, for this technology to be useful in modifying endothelial cell or smooth muscle cell function within the vessel wall, one must clearly understand the molecular basis for many complex phenomena, including those involving luminal thrombosis and proliferation of abluminal tissues. The potential value of genetic engineering to modify vessel wall and graft tissue will depend on future advances addressing these issues. Personalized molecular medicine will undoubtedly extend into the field of gene therapy and will revolutionize our treatment and prevention of disease.

SPECIALIZATION

The days of an individual doctor setting a forearm fracture, delivering a baby, and then performing an appendectomy are gone in modern society. Medicine is complex. The reality is that serious surgical diseases are best treated by those having special skills, despite concerns that fragmented care occurs with specialization. The following addresses are most germane to Vascular Surgery as a distinct discipline, with the author's very personal reaction attesting to the value of specialty care when he found himself as a patient.

7

THE AMERICAN BOARD OF VASCULAR SURGERY

This is the author's Society for Vascular Surgery's Presidential address, read before the 51st Annual Meeting on June 2, 1997, in Boston, Massachusetts. The education of surgeons was controversial at the time and the perceived need for a general education often seemed to trump the need to ensure the best of a specialty education. This is clearly reflected in the following dissertation.

Most of us have never had a chance to address their peers as I do today. I'm not sure just what measure of success brings anyone to this podium or how lasting the message from it may be, but I do march to a certain drum, which was no doubt instilled in me by my parents and teachers. As a teenager a motto on the wall of my high school locker room was "Winners don't quit, quitters don't win." I can still see the tile letters of this motto. There are many things I've never been a winner at, and in fact I'm not sure being the winner is so important, but I do believe that being a success is important—a success in your profession and, just as important, a success in your personal life, with your own faith, friends, and family. A year ago my daughter got Bill Rogers to autograph a running poster for me with the inscription "The race is not always for the swift, but for those that keep on running." I had just finished the 100th Boston Marathon. How true this statement has been for me—and how true it was for all of us during the arduous years of our training; during those long and difficult operations; and more recently during our dealings with others who would encroach upon our ability to care for our patients. To be a success often means to simply keep on going.

The scientific practice of vascular surgery is exceedingly complex, and combined with the intricacies of dealing with health-care provid-

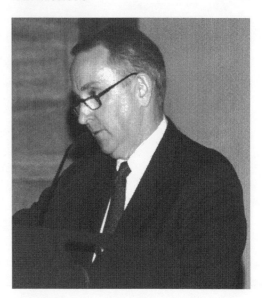

The author at the podium,
addressing the SVS mem-
bership in 1997

ers and well-intended social planners, as well as diverse distractions
from both our surgical and medical colleagues, challenges the simplest
of our efforts. My comments today address an important event in the
history of our discipline, the formation of the American Board of Vascular Surgery: the seeds of its evolution, the reactions to its inception,
and a reflection as to what this all means.

Development of a specialty in any field fosters greater in-depth
knowledge and advances a profession, but it carries the additional
caveat in medicine of enhancing patient care. Some believe that specialists can't render total care and that patients in general will be poorly
served by such specialists, who have fragmented the system. I don't
accept this tenet or its implication. Others believe that mediocre performance of subspecialty care by generalists is an increasing problem. I
do share their concern.

A few facts seem incontestable. First, extraordinary amounts of new
information have led many surgeons to specialize simply in order to
maintain basic competence in their clinical practices. Second, specialists undertaking greater numbers of specific procedures usually provide better outcomes. Third, although the generalist was by necessity
important because of inaccessible specialty care decades ago, contem-

porary information systems and more economical means of transportation have made specialized care available for most of society. This is not to discount those impoverished or uninsured individuals who have difficulty gaining access to any health-care providers be they generalists or specialists.

The evolution of the American Board of Vascular Surgery had its roots in our Societies more than 25 years ago. Jack Wylie in 1970 suggested that standards of excellence for vascular surgery could be reached by the establishment of specific residency training programs, and the need for this was echoed by Jack Cannon in 1971, who noted that lack of proper training and operations performed by occasional vascular surgeons did not serve patients well. During this same time period, James DeWeese, William Blaisdell, and John Foster had been appointed as a committee of the Inter-Society Commission for Heart Disease Resources. In 1972 they published a classic document on optimal training and practice standards in vascular surgery, including a recommendation that the American Board of Surgery and the American Board of Thoracic Surgery, or a sub-board of either or both boards, develop examinations in vascular surgery.

Over the next few years the issue of training and certification was discussed widely among members of our Societies, and in 1972 Keith Reemtsma and Jack Wylie submitted a resolution, approved by both Societies, recommending that the ABS issue certificates in vascular surgery. Both the American College of Surgeons and the American Surgical Association lent support to this and in 1973 Dr. Wylie presented his proposal to the American Board of Surgery, which approved his resolution in principle but asked for a more detailed proposal. Dr. Wylie presented his revised proposal to the ABS in 1974, yet the board was still not prepared to proceed with certification of vascular surgeons. Instead they established a standing committee to be known as the "Committee for Vascular Surgery."

The Committee for Vascular Surgery wasn't able to move the Board. No further action on Dr. Wylie's proposal was taken during the next year by the Board, nor was there any action following a second year. At that juncture, the Joint Council of the two vascular Societies appointed its own committee on vascular surgery training. The response of the American Board of Surgery one week after the establishment of our committee was that discussions of certification of vascular surgeons were premature and should not be considered at that time. Three years had been spent in developing guidelines for training programs, which were not acceptable to the ABS. Nevertheless, a year later these guidelines were accepted by the Residency Review Committee. This was remarkable.

This RRC training program proposal was forwarded to the Liaison Committee for Graduate Medical Education, but the proposal was tabled because of an objection from the American Board of Thoracic Surgery. Furthermore, the LCGME was not in a position to approve a training program for which there was no certificate, and the ABS was not about to provide one at that time.

At that point, in 1979, the Societies proposed their own committee to proceed with evaluation and accreditation of vascular surgery training programs, composed of Jack Wylie, Jim DeWeese, Sterling Edwards, Ed Garrett, and Jessie Thompson, the so-called "Program Evaluation and Endorsement Committee—the PEEC group." In 1980, perhaps because of this self-generated activity on behalf of the Vascular Societies, the American Board of Surgery and the American Board of Thoracic Surgery and their two corresponding Residency Review Committees changed their tact and unanimously approved the guidelines for training programs in vascular surgery. Final approval by all regulatory groups including the ABMS occurred in November 1982, more than a decade after the proposal had been initially developed by our Society leadership. In 1982 the first certifying examination was administered, and in 1984 the Residency Review Committee accredited its first training program.

At that time, in 1984, there was great concern expressed by the leadership of your Societies regarding a number of issues, including representation of vascular surgeons on the American Board of Surgery and the Residency Review Committee, as well as specific case numbers being required to allow individuals to sit for the certifying examination. Sound familiar? That was over 13 years ago. Not too different from today.

The designation of "special" qualifications on the ABS Certificate also proved to be a contentious issue. Many on the American Board of Surgery believed that this represented a unique certificate that did not solely relate to the surgeons' clinical performance of vascular procedures, but instead recognized their additional special contributions to the discipline of vascular surgery, including: research, publications and presentations, teaching of medical students and residents, academic appointments, as well as membership and participation in regional and national vascular Societies. Others, including many of the leaders of our Societies, believed that this devalued the purpose of the certificate, which was to recognize successful training in vascular surgery—training that was meant to improve patient care in later practice. The Board's interpretation of what "special" meant clearly made certification elusive to many individuals, including a number of you in this room, and gave the aura of elitism to the efforts of our predecessors. Transference of this action from the American Board of Surgery leadership to our Societies did not enhance our reputation among real-world practitioners, but we were not the culprits in this matter.

The purpose of my detailing these early happenings between the vascular surgery community and the American Board of Surgery is to establish the fact that difficulties in communicating and resolving differences of opinion between these groups did not arise during the past few years, but have been present since the earliest days of our specialty.

Having had 15 years' experience with formal ABMS recognized training programs in vascular surgery, it would seem logical to ask what impact these have had on patient care. After all, that's what we're supposed to be all about. On first pass, it appears that care is better, albeit seemingly provided by fewer but better trained surgeons. Two basic questions must be addressed. Will we continue to train sufficient numbers of surgeons to care for patients as we enter the next millennium? Will they provide quality care? My qualified answer is yes to both questions, but only if we and others change the way we train and the way we certify, as well as the way we practice.

The first issue I wish to call to your attention relates to numbers. If we attempt to ensure sufficient numbers of physicians to provide for care of patients with vascular disease, we must recognize certain limitations of our current training programs. This issue is compounded by the baby boomers as they enter our patient population, with an almost unbelievable 73% increase in those older than 65 years occurring from the year 2010 to 2030, and a resulting increase of operative interventions from 232 to 313 procedures per 100,000 population. If such were the case the total number of operations needed to be performed in 2020 would be 1,020,000. Remember that figure 1,020,000.

Vascular surgeons were responsible for approximately 51% of the total operations performed five years ago, and if the activities per surgeon remain unchanged, then 3,042 vascular surgeons would be required to provide for 51% of 1,020,000 operations needed in 2020, yet the product of our current training programs will provide only 2,370 of such surgeons. That's a shortfall of nearly 700 vascular surgeons! Given the length of training needed to enter practice we would be required to train nearly 30 additional fellows a year, starting now to meet these needs. This seems like a very large number and I am not advocating that we immediately increase our programs to meet this need. However, I might point out to you that this projection assumes that general surgeons will continue to also contribute as they have in the past, which does not appear likely. But just say they do; then in 2020 they will be responsible for approximately 150,000 operations, and Vascular surgeons will perform approximately 400,000 operations in that year. The total of 550,000 is unfortunately way short of the 1,020,000 operations required by society at that time. Who will provide the additional half-million procedures? General surgeons, given their own interests, malpractice costs, and limited hospital staff privileges, won't. The tenant that the small numbers of vascular operations performed by general surgeons today could well become smaller is quite logical, and places an even greater workload on the vascular surgery community.

Because the numbers required to train general surgeons in vascular procedures are mandated by RRC criteria, we as teachers are boxed in without sufficient operative cases available at many institutions to train additional vascular surgeons. This is unfortunate, because the data are clear that most general surgeons do not utilize their training experiences in vascular surgery to care for patients with vascular disease in their later careers. The American Board of Surgery has remained steadfast in their perception of the totally trained surgeon at the completion of residency being able to perform vascular surgery well. They may be able, but they don't do it in practice. This becomes a societal problem if we have the material to train but we don't produce a product to care for these patients. Even if you reduce societies' operative needs by 20 or 30%, which could occur with mandated changes in health care or introduction of new technology, such as endovascular therapies, we will still fall short in the number game.

Quality care is the second issue I wish to call to your attention. Data do not favor the occasional surgeon performing vascular surgery. Endarterectomy of the carotid artery is a good example. It is among the most common of vascular surgical procedures performed; the indications for it are reasonably well defined; the technical challenges of the procedure are not great; and many practitioners believe they are vested in the requisite skills to perform this procedure. Nevertheless, data document that those who perform fewer operations have much poorer outcomes than those who perform this procedure on a regular basis, and the latter are predominantly vascular surgeons, not general surgeons.

In the state of Iowa where there appeared to be an unacceptable high stroke rate following carotid endarterectomy, a careful audit of actual medical records for all 806 carotid endarterectomies performed on Medicare patients in 1994 revealed a combined cerebrovascular accident and mortality rate for procedures performed by Board-certified vascular surgeons of 5.2% compared to 8.4% for procedures performed by nonvascular surgeons. The 3.2% difference represents an incremental increase in stroke and death in excess of 60%. I would ask you the simple question whether it is reasonable for a patient to accept an added 3.2% risk of having a stroke or losing one's life just for the convenience of being treated by someone who believes that they are well trained in this procedure, compared to a vascular surgeon who has outcomes substantially better.

We are not talking about turf or egos and we shouldn't be talking about economics; we are talking about lives and the benefits of specialization as they relate to one of the most simple technical procedures in vascular surgery, certainly much less complex than the performance of an abdominal aortic aneurysmectomy or infrapopliteal bypass. Norman Hertzer was absolutely correct in his Presidential Address to us five years ago: results mean everything. Experiences such as that in Iowa do not favor treatment by the general surgeon. Either we need to train these surgeons differently or they need to practice differently.

The Strategic Planning group of your Societies (composed of the two Past Presidents, the two current Presidents, the two President-Elects, as well as the two Secretaries) met after last year's meeting, and considered how to establish a more forthright and effective dialogue with the American Board of Surgery and the Residency Review Committee in Surgery. We came to the conclusion that many issues facing patients and vascular surgeons in real-world practices were not going to be addressed simply by a continuing debate. In September 1996, the eight of us, (Drs. Smith, Veith, Goldstone, Baker, Abbott, Whittemore, Towne, and myself) proceeded with the incorporation of the American Board of Vascular Surgery. This action was carefully conceived with legal counsel and quiet input from many others. It was meant as a pre-emptive move. We own the name of the Board. The cost of creating this Board and its effect on our influence on American medicine were carefully weighed. We felt confident that this was the right thing to do, and the right time to do it.

Creation of the new Board was subsequently announced to the Executive Committee of the Program Directors in Vascular Surgery, the President of the Program Directors in General Surgery, the two vascular surgeons on the American Board of Surgery, the Chairman and Executive Director of the American Board of Surgery, and the Director of the American College of Surgeon, during sequential meetings on the same day in October 1996.

The reaction to our action might have been predicted. It caused considerable uneasiness among certain general surgeons. However, it has already resulted in a number of responses from the ABS and RRC addressing symptoms of our past inability to affect change, including: the option to recertify in general surgery, rather than having it as a man-datory requirement before recertification in vascular surgery; tabling by the Residency Review Committee, of the requirement for specific numbers of aortic cases to be performed by all general surgery trainees, which would have placed nearly a quarter of vascular surgery training programs in jeopardy; and the appointment of two vascular surgeons to the Residency Review Committee, and the anticipated appointment of an additional vascular surgeon to the American Board of Surgery, to be nominated by the Program Directors in Vascular Surgery. These actions have been a welcome respite, but they don't get at the root of our con-cerns, namely the trainee numbers and quality of care issues.

The American Board of Surgery missive of March 1997 penned by their Executive Director was not viewed favorably by your leadership. This document, sent to all 28,000 of you who are ABS certificate hold-ers, misinterprets and misrepresents the actions of the vascular surgery leadership. Dr. Robert Smith, my counterpart as President of the North American Chapter of the International Society for Cardiovascular Surgery, and myself, first met with the Chairman and Executive Director of the American Board of Surgery in October 1996 and clearly stated that we did not believe that the training of general surgeons in vascular surgery should be eliminated. We made this matter plentifully clear by stating that should the vascular communities' efforts to have a Board succeed, that a contractual agreement mandating the training of general surgeons in vascular surgery should exist for at least two decades.

How this could be interpreted to represent our wishing to cease training of general surgeons is beyond belief. To me, this is one of the most egregious faults in that communication, and although it may have been a defining moment for the Board's Executive Director it polarized much of the general surgery and vascular surgery communities. We have not gone as public in our response to the Board, but we have communicated directly to the Executive Director of the ABS, and have addressed a number of specific issues through correspondence from Cal Ernst to the Board. As you know Dr. Ernst was nominated to the ABS by our Joint Societies.

The vascular surgeons who represent your Societies are not intellectual terrorists. Our concerns are that lives are at stake, not reputations of organizations or the egos of their leadership. The American Board of Surgery through their recent communication revealed an exceptional talent for making vascular surgeons look petty, but in the rush to condemn us, two things were forgotten: our surgical trainees and our patients. The hubris that the American Board of Surgery should be applauded for being the arbiter and caretaker of vascular surgery's future is not borne out by their actions of the past 25 years.

On the other hand we should really not be at odds with the ABS. We need a solution, not hierarchical dictates from anyone, be they from ourselves, other surgical organizations, or the American Board of Surgery. But time is not a luxury in this effort. Given the changing face of medical practice, indolence may be the greatest threat to our specialty. We will not keep our vigor and coherence if we are too timid to engage, to challenge, or to inspire.

In our last public communication to those in our Societies, we asked for your support at pursuing our request to establish a primary Board within the American Board of Medical Specialists. It was signed by the Councils of both Societies and the Association of Program Directors in Vascular Surgery. I doubt that few times in our history has such unanimous resolve been publicly expressed. We received a total of 1,276 replies of which 11% were undecided. Among those rendering an opinion 906 favored our actions and 231 did not. Thus, 80% of those with an opinion favored the formation of the American Board of Vascular Surgery. Perhaps most important were the responses from questionnaires sent to the 815 members holding ABS certificates in vascular surgery: 767 replied, with only 48 failing to reply. Among Board certified vascular surgeons who replied, 644 favored our action. Only 60 disapproved. Thus, among Board certified vascular surgeons rendering an opinion, 91% favored pursuing recognition of the American Board of Vascular Surgery. This Board certified group was decidedly younger than the noncertified respondents, and are likely to be the future voice of our Societies.

The scope of this effort has been politically tedious if not daunting. Although we meet all of the ABMS criteria to become a primary Board, throughout the discussions by the eight who founded the American Board of Vascular Surgery on your behalf, we have considered the wisdom of proposing that it be an ABMS Conjoint Board rather than a Primary Board. From an operational perspective a Conjoint Board is almost identical to a Primary Board.

The difference between a Primary Board and Conjoint Board is that the Directors of the Conjoint Board are appointed by two sponsoring Boards, which in our case we believe should be the American Board of Surgery and the American Board of Thoracic Surgery. The thoracic surgeons have a great deal at stake in what we do regarding further specialization and training, in that 35% of their certificate holders currently perform 50 or more vascular procedures a year. Appointments by these two boards to the American Board of Vascular Surgery directorship would come from nominations from Societies such as ours, the Program Directors in Vascular Surgery, and the Regional Vascular Societies.

The conduct of a Conjoint Board must be in concert with the missions of the sponsoring boards, yet the day-to-day operations would not be hindered by the reoccurring problems that have plagued us during the past quarter century with those presently responsible for controlling our training programs and certifying us as practitioners.

Our goal should not be to expend considerable energy on political polemic. However, if we don't address the issues as to whether we will have enough vascular surgeons properly trained to care for patients as we enter the next century, then we will have been derelict to our profession and society.

The American Board of Surgery faces many difficulties, only one of which is the challenge that has been laid before it by your Societies leadership. They must recognize that specialization will invariably cause some degree of fragmentation, and that unfortunately certification in the real world provides improved opportunities for physicians as they attempt to gain hospital credentials.

It may not be my place, but I personally believe that the American Board of Surgery should seriously consider restructuring the manner with which it appoints its Directors, such that they are elected so as to more likely represent the various special components of surgery rather than various popular leaders of clinical and academic societies. It would also be my personal advice that they consider surgical oncology, hepatobiliary and gastrointestinal surgery, critical care and trauma, transplantation, and endocrine surgery in a different venue than currently exists, such that these subspecialties will have a greater responsibility and, most importantly, the authority to define how surgeons are trained and certified in their areas of expertise.

Like many of my predecessors, I believe that vascular surgery should continue to be a part of the training of the general surgeon, but not as a primary component. Furthermore, because of the distinct body of knowledge encompassing vascular surgery, and practice issues related to better patient care, the vascular surgery community should be respected for having evolved to the point where a greater degree of independence as a Conjoint Board deserves support.

Your leadership has met with many individuals and organizations in the past nine months and has concluded this year with three commitments.

First, we believe that the Curriculum and Conjoint Data Committees, developed by us in recent discussions with the American Board of Surgery and others, should continue their work with a definitive report from these Committees expected by the October 1997 Joint Council Meeting.

Second, we will defer until February 1998 submission of our application to the Liaison Committee of the American Board of Medical Specialists to become a Primary Board. The completed application will remain unpublicized in our hands, but there is a time frame.

Third, we will request support for a Conjoint Board from our colleagues on the American Board of Surgery and the American Board of Thoracic Surgery. The logic in creating a Conjoint Board is solid and benefits would be derived by both organizations in supporting the vascular surgery community in this action.

Closure on this effort will likely be measured in years, not weeks or months. We have the support of many nonsurgeons in the American Board of Medical Specialists. We need the respect of many surgical organizations, including the American Surgical Association and American College of Surgeons. We are not elitists, and we're not the enemy. In fact, we're a lot like everyone else: we care about the Discipline of Surgery, and our patients.

It has been said that a single conversation across the table with a wise man is worth hours and days in the library. During the past year as your President, I have had many conversations with individuals who have given me great insight into myself and into our discipline. The seven others who have had conversations with me during the establishment of the American Board of Vascular Surgery are remarkable individuals. It is important that you recognize just what they've done on your behalf. We will need the help of all of you as we proceed—be you a practitioner in the trenches or an academic, an active participant in the Societies, or not. You are all part of our Discipline and we need you.

That we should be so inbred, isolated, and reactionary, that we forget who we are, would be a travesty. We are vascular surgeons. Our discipline is no longer in its adolescence. It has lost its innocence and has become a mature specialty with major obligations to Society. We should not fail in these obligations.

8

FINITE ELEMENTS: A MATTER OF TIME

This address represents the 13th Richard E. Fry Lecture, which was read before the 58th Clinical Meeting of the Frederick A. Coller Surgical Society on September 22, 2012, in Annapolis, Maryland. It was meant to reflect on serious illnesses and the role of physicians and surgeons in providing the best care possible. It represents a very personal statement about the author's health.

The invitation to deliver this address is a singular honor. I've been fortunate to have had the bully pulpit at this meeting twice before, first in 1995 as President when I spoke of "Mentorship," and then in 1997 when I spoke about "Yesteryear and Yesterday," a biographic sketch of Drs. Frederick Coller and Milton Bryant, given as a replacement of Milt's presidential address following his tragic death a few months earlier in an automobile accident. My address today is personal. I hope you will understand.

Dick Fry was remarkably bright, an excellent surgeon, caring husband, and devoted young father who was robbed of life at too young of an age. I knew Dick best as a medical student when Marvin Kirsh first introduced him to Michelle. Both Nancy and I attended their wedding. To say they were a happy and gifted young couple would be an understatement. The world was theirs—until his cough proved not to be bronchitis. It was cancer. Cancer is an illness that may leave you defenseless, even if you are a doctor. Dick had done all the right things. He just was unable to add more time to his existence, for his wife and kids, for his parents and brother, and for his patients. That should be a palpable loss to all of us.

It is often hard to talk candidly of one's professional and personal life, but let me try to share some of my own, private feelings about both. I want to speak about two things we often don't talk about at our annual meeting: conflict amongst our profession and personal loss of control. Just so you don't get the wrong idea, let me tell you this presentation is about the best of care.

First, let me address what I mean by the best of care. A surgeon's life is different; anesthetized patients can't negotiate with us and it's difficult to reverse what you've done with your hands after the fact. Whatever we start in the operating room we have to finish in a reasonable period of time. We don't have the luxury to think things over and adjust our care the next day. Time is not on our side. If a patient deserves your best when they're asleep and have placed their lives in your hands, then what else matters? I think not much. You certainly wouldn't want someone caring for you who has had little experience with a given operation or whose mind is more on convincing themselves and others that they can do the big cases. If you were the patient with a so-called big case, you'd want the best from a well-trained experienced surgeon. My initial admiration for surgeons was for those who looked like they could do everything, even if they fell a little short at some things. I no longer feel that way. I simply don't believe that if you know the anatomy, can tie a square knot really fast, and know a lot about the disease, that you have license to operate. Some believe the "jack of all trades" approach to surgical care is acceptable. You know the argument that we need the "generalist" for the rural areas, but how about New York, Chicago, and other populated areas where 95% of our citizens live? I don't buy this and neither should you.

I would like to share with you two disparate scenarios about best of care: one involving Dick Kraft and the other Mary Travers.

The first was Dick Kraft's well thought out Presidential Address at the 1975 Coller meeting. It must have been one of the earliest comparisons of individual staff competencies by a Department chair. He identified outliers regarding critical elements of surgical care, like blood loss during a procedure and time in the OR. To conclude that some of the outliers shouldn't be surgeons might be an overkill, but nevertheless I'm not sure I would want them to operate on me. The outliers and their close-by peers might better do what they do well and stay the course, not operating beyond their training or talent, but referring more difficult cases to someone else who could offer a better outcome, even someone in a different practice group or another hospital. Now there's a thought—actually putting the patient's welfare first. I was three years out of my residency when I heard these words from Dick. I have not forgotten them.

The second scenario occurred some three decades later in 2005, when Nancy and I heard Peter, Paul and Mary perform in Philadelphia. Mary Travers had just completed extensive treatment for advanced cancer, and after chemotherapy and whole body radiation she had received a marrow transplant. Her comment to a very appreciative audience was, "If you're really sick, find a good doctor and a good hospital, even if it's inconvenient." She had it right. I always believed that for the individual patient surgical specialization is better medical care, even if it's not at arm's reach.

These two experiences are lead-ins to my speaking to you about specialization in the practice of medicine. In another time eons and eons ago, life probably evolved from the generation of organic compounds in a primordial sea of simple finite elements. And that took time. As evolution progressed so did the survival skills and sophistication of all advanced life on this earth. Not every species survived. Similarly, specialization in medicine has evolved from one generation to another generation, and some practices have disappeared. These changes in medicine have not always been pain-free or peaceful. And not all fields of medicine have survived. I would like to tell you about the evolution of the specialty held by Dick Fry and six of the last seven Coller Presidents: the specialty of vascular surgery.

Vascular surgery as we know it was conceived nearly 75 years ago. It was followed by the stress of being a subordinate subspecialty for decades—doing something in the OR because it made sense, even when no one had ever written or talked about it, and pain with its birthing as a mature specialty in the 1970s existed when terrible vascular surgical outcomes in patients were being seen throughout the country. Clearly, the training of many general surgeons who were about to undertake arterial reconstructions in their practice was inadequate in those days.

Recognition of the need for improved training first resulted in a set of proposed training standards being submitted to the American Board of Surgery and American Board of Thoracic Surgery by a group of senior vascular surgeons led by Jim DeWeese in 1972. From the community of vascular surgeons' perspective this proposal was not about their making more money, controlling hospital resources, or building their collective ego. It was about providing society with the future surgeons who would provide better care.

The American Board of Surgery wanted no part of this and responded in a very terse statement that they were "not prepared to proceed." They had defined the subject as a "turf" issue. The year was 1972.

Subsequently a committee for Vascular Surgery evolved, led by Jack Wylie from San Francisco. Ignoring the Board's rebuff, they created a set of unofficial guidelines that were voluntarily offered to programs around the country. Under the direction of the nation's two vascular societies, these educational efforts morphed into what was known as the PEEC group, an acronym for Program Evaluation and Endorsement Committee. By 1979 it was all about training, and many outstanding surgery residents were eager to participate. This voluntary action was very successful, and became a de facto threat to the American Board of Surgery—after all they were being beat at the very game they were supposed to be responsible for.

Subsequently, in 1980, the ABS and ABTS approved guidelines similar to the PEEC ones.

Then in 1982, when Bill Fry, a past Coller Society president, was the Chairman of the American Board of Surgery, this organization offered a certificate of "Special Qualifications in General Vascular Surgery." The certificate was controversial and the elitism associated with the word "special" was offensive to practicing surgeons in the private sector. The Board attributed this to the elite nature of the vascular surgery community. Such was nonsense. The Board simply wanted the certificate to be in the hands of a limited number of highly specialized vascular surgeons—who, by the way, in order to be certified had to have documented credentials in participating in surgical societies, educating trainees, or publishing papers—for whatever that had to do with clinical competence at the operating table! The first certifying exam was given to 14 sitting members of the American Board of Surgery, including some who had not done any vascular cases in years. It was an uncomfortable start, but it was a start.

The first certificate, number 1, was appropriately given to Jack Wylie, and it was Bill Fry who signed his certificate. The initial 400 or so certificates were mostly grandfathered in. Formal training programs were in the mill.

By 1984 the American Board of Medical Specialists, the ABMS, who have authority over the individual Specialty Boards like the American Board of Surgery regarding their issuance of new certificates, had approved the separate training of vascular surgeons, over the objections of the American Board of Surgery. Vascular surgery was born by a near unanimous vote by other ABMS Boards, who were disenchanted with the American Board of Surgery's unwillingness to allow osteopaths to sit for their exam, even if they had completed a Board approved training program. For years other specialties had accepted osteopaths into their programs and allowed them to become certified. So those voting in favor of our existence perhaps didn't like us as much as they disliked the American Board of Surgery.

After being born of ill-respected parents who themselves considered Vascular Surgery to be an errant stepchild, things got worse. The American Board of Surgery declared for the first time they needed quantitative data and numerical targets for the general surgery trainees to be eligible to sit for their Board exam: 44 major arterial reconstructions were the minimum needed for each graduating resident. It's interesting that many other complex procedures done solely by general surgeons were not assigned a quota number. As well intended as it may have been, only a little more than half the training programs could comfortably meet the vascular numbers, and it was clear that adding a fellowship in vascular surgery would only detract from the general surgery trainee's ability to meet their quota, and such could potentially put the general surgery program in jeopardy. So you guessed it—vascular training independent of general surgery was in disfavor at that time. That was in the 1980s.

And pettiness arose. The American Board of Surgery issued certificates that were purposely smaller in size than the certificate most of us held after completing a general surgery training program and passing the Board's examination. No other Board was issuing "small" certificates. On the table the ABS even had discussions about having a simple stamp that could be placed on the existing general surgery certificate or applied to one of the newer smaller certificates every 10 years when you recertified. This behavior was rather weird.

This conflict continued to smolder for a little more than a decade, until 1996 when Frank Veith, who preceded me as the President of the Society for Vascular Surgery, spoke about evolution in the practice of vascular surgery. The movement toward the independence for vascular surgery had become a subject of conversation.

Later that year, Robert Smith and I as the sitting presidents of the two national vascular societies oversaw the legal incorporation of the American Board of Vascular Surgery. The founding group encompassed the Executive Councils of the Society for Vascular Surgery and North American Chapter of the International Society for Cardiovascular Surgery. Our intent was to seek ABMS approval as an independent Board.

The political nature of the quest for independence intensified when a manifesto regarding the rationale for the establishment of the American Board of Vascular Surgery, signed by the leaders of both national organizations, as well as the Association of Program Directors in Vascular Surgery, was published in *The Journal of Vascular Surgery*. That was in 1997.

This was followed by my presidential address before the Society for Vascular Surgery, which was a direct challenge to the existing attitude and utterances of the American Board of Surgery. A lot of posturing was going on. But a "real" Board approved by the ABMS and not simply a rogue Board, which it clearly was at the time, would prove a daunting task.

Over the next five years we laid the groundwork to obtain ABMS approval, and in 2002 we petitioned the ABMS to become a specialty distinct from general surgery. Jack Cronenwett, another Coller Society member, and I joined Frank Veith at a formal presentation before the Liaison Committee, accompanied with a voluminous application. The criteria to become such a Board were tightly proscribed in their Reference Handbook. Our application included specific documentation as to how Vascular Surgery met each of the criteria of a certifying Board, as defined in Section IV of their own published criteria for Board eligibility.

We received notice in a letter dated two days later that our petition was rejected. Within a week we asked to be informed of the specific reasons for the rejection. We were rebuffed again without any details regarding the very criteria for which we believed we had been judged— and had allegedly not met. This was maddening.

SPECIAL COMMUNICATION

The American Board of Vascular Surgery: Rationale for its formation

January 3, 1997

Dear SVS and ISCVS-NA Members:

Considerable advances in the diagnosis and treatment of patients with vascular disease have occurred during recent decades. A major portion of the new knowledge and innovative techniques that contributed to these advances has come from vascular surgeons. The specialty of Vascular Surgery has evolved into a distinct entity concerned with the pathogenesis, diagnosis, and treatment of arterial, venous, and lymphatic diseases.

The leadership of the Society for Vascular Surgery (SVS), International Society for Cardiovascular Surgery-North American Chapter (ISCVS-NA), and Association of Program Directors in Vascular Surgery (APDVS) believe that two principles must be at the forefront of our organizations' missions. The first is to provide constant improvement in the efficient and excellent care of patients with vascular disease. The second is the development and maintenance of the best means for training professionals to care for patients with vascular disease.

The governing bodies of General Surgery, in particular the American Board of Surgery (ABS) and the Residency Review Committee in Surgery (RRC-S), have had a profound impact on the training, certification, practice, and status of Vascular Surgery. Over the past decade, it has become apparent that there are problems in the relationship between these governing bodies and Vascular Surgery. These problems have been transmitted to your leadership from practicing vascular surgeons and those who have the responsibility to teach future generations of vascular surgeons. Although the intent of this communication is not to be inflammatory, many issues remain

Correspondence to: American Board of Vascular Surgery, Thirteen Elm St., Manchester, MA 01944-1314.
J Vasc Surg 1997;25:411-3.
Copyright © 1997 by The Society for Vascular Surgery and International Society for Cardiovascular Surgery, North American Chapter.
0741-5214/97/$5.00 + 0 24/6/80103

unresolved. For instance, it seems unnecessary for a vascular surgeon who cares only for vascular surgery patients and who does not otherwise perform general surgery to be required by the ABS to recertify in General Surgery before being eligible for the examination for Re-Certification with Added Qualifications in General Vascular Surgery. We acknowledge that it is reasonable for a surgeon to be examined in General Surgery as well as Vascular Surgery, if that surgeon's practice ...

JOURNAL OF VASCULAR SURGERY
Volume 25, Number 2   American Board of Vascular Surgery

For the SVS Council:	For the ISCVS-NA Executive Council:	For the APDVS Executive Committee:
James C. Stanley, M.D.* *President*	Robert B. Smith III, M.D.* *President*	Jonathan B. Towne, M.D.* *President*
William M. Abbott, M.D.* *President Elect*	William H. Baker, M.D.* *President Elect*	Robert W. Hobson, II, M.D. *President Elect*
Jonathan B. Towne, M.D.* *Secretary*	Anthony D. Whittemore, M.D.* *Secretary*	Jack L. Cronenwett, M.D. *Secretary-Treasurer*
Christopher K. Zarins, M.D. *Treasurer*	Alexander W. Clowes, M.D. *Treasurer*	John W. Hallett, M.D. *Councillor*
Jack L. Cronenwett, M.D. *Recorder*	William H. Pearce, M.D. *Recorder*	Joseph L. Mills, M.D. *Councillor*
Thomas J. Fogarty, M.D. *Past President*	Jerry Goldstone, M.D.* *Past President*	John J. Ricotta, M.D. *Councillor*
Norman R. Hertzer, M.D. *Past President*	Robert B. Rutherford, M.D. *Past President*	Christopher K. Zarins, M.D. *Councillor*
Frank J. Veith, M.D.* *Past President*	Ronald J. Stoney, MD *Past President*	John M. Porter, M.D. *Past President*
Bruce J. Brener, M.D. *ACS Representative*	Norman R. Hertzer, M.D. *ACS Representative*	* Directors of the American Board of Vascular Surgery

The ABSV manifesto, 1997

We subsequently appealed the decision to the AMA, one of the organizations responsible for appointing members to the Liaison Committee. Just consider the response in their reply to us: "No vote was taken on each of the individual criteria…" and "Therefore, no formal record exists of which of the criteria formed the basis for the denial. Due to this, there is no way to provide you with the information that you request." It was almost surreal to read that this public body had no formal records relating to the meeting's sole purpose of hearing our proposal, or the specific basis of our rejection. However, we did not go away.

AMERICAN BOARD OF MEDICAL SPECIALTIES®
1007 Church Street, Suite 404   Evanston, Illinois 60201-5913   847/491-9091
FAX: 847/328-3596
http://www.abms.org

December 20, 2002

James C. Stanley, MD
Professor of Surgery
Head, Section of Vascular Surgery
University of Michigan
1500 E. Medical Center Drive
2210 Taubman
Ann Arbor, MI 48109

Dear Dr. Stanley:

The Liaison Committee for Specialty Boards (LCSB) convened a meeting to review the application by the American Board of Vascular Surgery for approval as an ABMS Examining Board in Medical Specialties on December 18, 2002.

The committee has asked me to extend its sincere appreciation to yourself, and Doctors Cronenwett and Veith, for coming to Chicago to provide an overview of your application and to clarify issues for the LCSB during its deliberations.

Following a careful discussion and consideration, the LCSB has requested that I notify you that the application of the American Board of Vascular Surgery to become a new Examining Board in Medical Specialties was denied. This conclusion was based on a careful and extensive review of the application, the information provided at the hearings and the letters received regarding this application. This decision was in accord with the requirements of "the Eleventh Revision for Essentials for Approval of Examining Boards of Medical Specialties."

Under section V.H. The American Board of Vascular Surgery may file a formal appeal. This appeal must be written and provided to the Secretary of the LCSB within 6 months of your notification of a negative decision by the LCSB.

Sincerely yours,

Stephen H. Miller, MD, MPH
Secretary LCSB

Cc.   James L. Borland, Jr., MD
        David L. Nahrwold, MD   Barbara Barzansky, PhD

G:\COMMITTEES\Lcsb\AB of Vasc Surgery\Stanleyltr12-18-02.doc

The ABMS rejection letter without specific cause being noted, 2002

December 26, 2002

Stephen H. Miller, M.D., M.P.H.
Secretary, Liaison Committee for Specialty Boards
American Board of Medical Specialties
1007 Church Street, Suite 404
Evanston, IL 60201-5913

Dear Dr. Miller:

This letter is written in response to your communication of December 20, 2002 stating that the Liaison Committee for Specialty Boards had denied the application of the American Board of Vascular Surgery to become an ABMS Examining Board in Medical Specialties.

We would appreciate being informed of the specific shortcomings of this application in reference to the "Essentials for Approval of Examining Boards of Medical Specialties". Such information will be necessary for the American Board of Vascular Surgery to determine the appropriateness of an appeal or reapplication at a later time.

Sincerely yours,

James C. Stanley, M.D.
Chairman, American Board of Vascular Surgery

cc: James L. Borland, Jr., MD
       David R. Nahrwold, MD
       Barbara Barzansky, PhD

The ABVS request for specific information, 2002.

AMERICAN BOARD OF MEDICAL SPECIALTIES®

1007 Church Street, Suite 404   Evanston, Illinois 60201-5913   847/491-9091
FAX: 847/328-3596
http://www.abms.org

December 30, 2002

James C. Stanley, MD
Professor of Surgery
Head, Section of Vascular Surgery
University of Michigan
1500 E. Medical Center Drive
2210 Taubman
Ann Arbor, MI 48109

Dear Dr. Stanley:

I am unable to provide more specific shortcomings of the application of the American Board of Vascular Surgery. The LCSB decision was based on a totality of criteria elucidated in the Eleventh Revision of Essentials for Approval of Examining Boards in Medical Specialties, Section IV Criteria for Approval of New Examining Boards.

Sincerely yours,

Stephen H. Miller, MD, MPH
Secretary LCSB

Cc.   James L. Borland, Jr., MD
      David L. Nahrwold, MD
      Barbara Barzansky, PhD

The ABMS response without specifics, 2002

78

American Medical Association
Physicians dedicated to the health of America

September 23, 2003

James C. Stanley, MD
Chairman
American Board of Vascular Surgery
221 West Walton
Chicago, IL 60610

Dear Dr. Stanley:

This is in response to your letter to the Executive Officers of the American Medical Association (AMA) requesting information about the reasons for the denial by the Liaison Committee for Specialty Boards (LCSB) of the application for recognition from the American Board of Vascular Surgery (ABVS). As you know, the AMA representatives to the LCSB are members of the Council on Medical Education, so your letter was referred to the Council for a response.

In discussing your request with its LCSB representatives, the Council determined that the vote to deny the application of the ABVS was a global one. No vote was taken on each of the individual criteria in the "Essentials for the Approval of Examining Boards in Medical Specialties." Therefore, no formal record exists of which of the criteria formed the basis for the denial. Due to this, there is no way to provide you with the information that you request.

Sincerely,

Michael D. Maves, MD, MBA
Executive Vice President, CEO

Emmanuel G. Cassimatis, MD
Chair, Council on Medical Education

cc: Board of Directors, ABVS
       Stephen H. Miller, MD, MPH

The AMA response noting no formal record of the rejection criteria exists, 2003

Shortly thereafter, in 2003 at a meeting in Philadelphia at the American Board of Surgery offices, a group of leaders from the major organizations involved in this political hassle met to discuss a primary certificate for vascular surgery, and a few months later the American Board of Surgery made a significant breakthrough with the establishment of this certificate—a certificate that could be gained by trainees independent of their having to first complete a general surgery residency. This represented much of what we had wished to achieve at the start in 1996.

The Primary Certificate in Vascular Surgery, finally approved in 2006, was available to those successfully completing their specialty training by a number of paths. Most importantly it included the establishment of a five-year integrated residency in Vascular Surgery, allowing medical students to begin their training directly after graduation, like orthopedics, otolaryngology, urology, or neurosurgery. This concept, initially proposed by Jack Cronenwett, was first initiated in 2007 at three institutions: Dartmouth, the University of Pittsburgh, and the University of Michigan. It did not void the continued opportunity to enter a vascular fellowship for individuals completing their five-year general surgery residency, but it was a breakthrough advance.

The existing female gender distribution before 2007 did not favor women entering Vascular Surgery training programs. At that time only five years ago, when the integrated program first started, only 27% of general surgery residents were women, and general surgery residents were the only talent pool from which vascular surgery fellows could arise. In fact, in those days only 20% of vascular surgery trainees were women. The new five-year programs made it possible for the more than half of this country's medical classes who are women to entertain being a vascular surgeon without the preamble of general surgery training. Given this opportunity, more than half of our trainees at Michigan are women. They are a remarkably talented group of whom the faculty are very proud to have in the ranks.

Even though the numbers have improved for those entering a vascular fellowship after their general surgery training, there still are some traditional programs following general surgery training that don't fill. That's not true of the five-year residencies.

The integrated five-year programs were inaugurated in 2007, and two of the first three—Dartmouth's and Michigan's —were headed up by Coller members, whose trainees, for the first time, were supervised by the vascular surgery program director, not the general surgery residency director. There are now 27 of these programs among the 114 total vascular surgery programs. Most extraordinarily, currently greater than half of those trainees in the five-year programs nationwide are women. So here we are in 2012—out of a very rich heritage of general surgery, vascular surgery emerged.

It has added to the dictum of what "best" is: it's not only the right operation at the right time for the right patient—it's by the right surgeon. Further specialization will be inevitable. I should be so bold as to suggest to many of the young in this hall that the rich primordial sea of surgery likely has other residual specialties in the process of being born to improve care. I hope some of you find the leadership to bring these other specialties to life. In addressing this political morass of Board issues, what I really want you to hear is that specialization is important to advance clinical science and improve patient care. Those that stubbornly refuse to recognize the value of expert care need a little more intellectual honesty and a little more personal responsibility—trying to do everything should not get you a medal and referring a patient to another practitioner is not a sin. They may not remember it, but most doctors made a commitment to this when they recited the Hippocratic Oath as they became physicians.

I practice on a medical campus today that is a good place for patients to receive their care. That came home to me in spades in May 2011. For more than 18 months, after decades of good health, I became a poster child for the ads on TV of the guy that missed the baseball game's triple because he was in the stadium's bathroom. I had had kidney stones 25 years earlier but I never had a urinary tract infection and didn't have to get up at night to urinate; my prostate gland was fine. In fact I was in great shape until I developed uninhibited bladder contractions. You know, I really had to hurry to the john to keep from soiling myself. I never did wet my pants, but after a year I was wearing Depends and carried spares with me. I had had cystoscopy years earlier and was told I likely had mild prostatitis from a stone that decades earlier had been stuck in my prostatic urethra for a day before it passed. There was nothing like dumping a few ml of urine into my paper underwear in the middle of a long operation or as I was chairing a meeting with the University President and the sitting Chair of the Board of Regents at the table. Those times didn't give me much confidence that all was well. At a subsequent social event I complained to a senior urologist that this didn't make a lot of sense, and five days later my suspicion that all was not well was borne out.

I had extensive bladder cancer, superficial urothelial carcinoma involving the vast majority of my bladder with extensions into my prostatic urethra and both ureters. Not a great thing to have and I had no idea if it had spread further—a sure death knell if such were the case. In the week after the diagnosis was made I became a student of urologic data, consulting with the Chair at Sloan Memorial in New York and the Head of Urology at MD Anderson, with whom I had previously operated with. I would have been out of Ann Arbor in a flash if someone had a few percent better outcomes elsewhere. I elected to be treated at the University of Michigan only after being told by these individuals that Michigan had an extraordinarily gifted surgeon there who I should consult—someone I didn't even know but a lot of others did. I met Khaled Hafez on a Tuesday. No nonsense—and an aggressive technician—that's what I wanted. I couldn't have cared less about his personality; I was going to be asleep when the chips were down. The next Monday I underwent a six-hour radical cancer operation—cystectomy and prostatectomy, and an ileal loop—but no muscle invasion and all 22 nodes were negative. That translates into a 70 to 75% cure. Not perfect, but who was I to object.

I was lucky and I had a good surgeon, actually not the one who had initially been suggested to me—a well-known good person, but a face-man who had the academic title but not the inner reputation of one who you might want to operate on you when you're asleep and defenseless. I wonder where he might have ranked on Dick Kraft's list. I had no hesitation in deciding who would treat me, and let me remind you that a radial cystectomy in the best reported series from premiere institutions carries a 4% mortality and a 25 to 30% major complication rate. Complex high-risk procedures like mine should not be done by the occasional surgeon just because an ABMS Board has granted that person a certificate.

This was obviously a life-altering happening for me. But here I am— no bladder, but a loop of bowel and two kidneys—and no tumor. It is perhaps fitting that on October 16th this year, my urologist will be recognized as one of three University of Michigan Clinicians of the Year. He made a difference. I had judged him on his technical expertise, and yet he had an unbelievably compassionate and caring personality. I'd build a statue for him, and my wife would like to adopt him. Hear me clearly: my greatest admiration and respect goes to those who operate on an anesthetized fellow human being and don't miss a stroke.

My professional life has been full, and my days spent at the Cardiovascular Center have been a fantasy: from groundbreaking, to its formal dedication, to today—a proven wonderful place to be busy helping others.

But my illness and convalescence was not so busy, and it gave me time to think about where I'd been and realize how fortunate I was to find myself in an environment that had grown with society's needs since my early days as a medical student in 1960

Three special Coller members made my early surgical education a pure joy. Bill DeWeese was a quiet and consummate gentleman. My rotation on his private service as a senior medical student became a tipping point in my life a year later during my internship at Philadelphia General Hospital. I had been accepted into Michigan's Internal Medicine Residency, but three months into my internship the value of that experience was the reason I called back to Ann Arbor and asked if I could be considered for a position in the surgery residency. They accepted me and my life was better for it.

Then there was Cal Ernst, who taught me what hard work meant. And Cal taught me how to write a clean simple sentence—a great investment, for decades after we first worked together, we became editors together of *The Journal of Vascular Surgery*. And of course there was Dick Fry's father, Bill, who was a legend as an educator; he pushed me to move along in the operating room, and served as an important role model as I became involved in the national vascular community. All three also gave me the understanding that you can't always have it your own way. You can't always be in control, and when you can't be in control, no matter what the issue is, find someone who knows what they know. Time counts.

For years as I was growing up we had a poster in our home above a study desk. Its message is as relevant today as it was a half-century ago.

He who knows not, but knows not that he knows not: IGNORE HIM
He who knows not, and knows that he knows not: TEACH HIM
He who knows, but knows not that he knows: AWAKE HIM, and
He who knows, and knows that he knows: FOLLOW HIM

I've lived with six Deans, two interim Deans, four Vice Presidents for Medical Affairs, and four Surgical Chairmen. In some sense I've followed all of them—each has added to my realizing what is important and what is not. The fact is that being a Michigan surgeon has brought a deep satisfaction to me every day and has shown me that my life has had meaning.

And, of course, I'd like to hang around a little longer, with a peace of mind that sometimes eludes busy surgeons. Life is profoundly valuable to all of us. In recent years with what extra time I can eke out of the day I've found a rewarding calm in creative writing—you know, no hypotheses to be proven or conclusions to be drawn. My having spent time with the Iowa Writers' group has allowed me to venture into intellectual and emotional territories I never thought possible.

And at the end of the day music has entered my busy existence.

Music has given Nancy and me a chance to spend time with some of the most talented people I would ever have dreamed would be part of my world. The likes of Yo-Yo Ma, Wynton Marsalis, or Valery Gergiev have revealed a rhythm of life that has made me appreciate the importance of artistic creativity. I've admitted before that I'm a bit of a groupie around most creative artists; they've helped me become a better listener and observer of humankind for the moments spent with them.

My family—there at the beginning and at the end of the day, have brought relevance to my life more than anything else, and have made me realize what a wonderful world this is. Nancy and I have been blessed with three wonderful children, Tim, Jeff, and Sarah, all married to neat spouses, all healthy and wise beyond our greatest hopes. And our four cool grandchildren, Annie, Teddy, Charlie, and Lauren, who possess inquisitiveness, energy, and laughter that has no boundaries bring joy to our lives.

Nancy, my college sweetheart, was by far and away the best of my growing up as an undergraduate student, and she was the ballast of my days in medical school following our marriage in 1961. Nancy has been my comforter, confessor, companion, and love for more than a half-century. She is the glue that has kept me together. I'm very lucky to be at her side.

Life's been good to me. So be it for you.

HISTORICAL NOTES

These two addresses reflect the author's life-long professional association with renal artery diseases and renovascular hypertension: the first being an overview of the national scene during the latter half of the 20th century, and the second depicting the rich heritage of the University of Michigan in this field of medicine.

9

SURGICAL TREATMENT OF RENOVASCULAR
HYPERTENSION: A HISTORY

This address was presented as the David M. Hume Memorial Lecture at the 25th Annual Meeting of the Society for Clinical Vascular Surgery on March 14, 1997, in Naples, Florida. It reflected the widespread contributions of many scientists and clinicians throughout the United States to our understanding of renovascular hypertension. The presentation in expanded form was published in Am J Surg 174:102–10, 1997. A second version of this address emphasizing the disease's underlying pathophysiology was presented as the I. S. Ravdin Lecture in the Basic Sciences at the 88th Clinical Congress of the American College of Surgeons on October 9, 2002, in San Francisco, California.

The contemporary surgical treatment of renovascular hypertension centers on the accomplishments of many laboratory and clinical scientists. This dissertation is a synopsis of the considerable advances that have led to the effective surgical treatment of renal artery occlusive disease in the United States.

The seminal contribution that established the relevance of a renal artery stenosis to arterial hypertension was made by Harry Goldblatt, MD, at the Western Reserve University. Goldblatt's classic canine experiments, first published in 1934, documented sustained hypertension following reductions in renal artery blood flow caused by the gradual closure of an adjustable vascular clamp about the renal artery. The hypertensive state in these animals resolved rapidly following removal of the affected kidney. This confirmed, beyond any doubt, the relationship between renal artery occlusive lesions and hypertension.

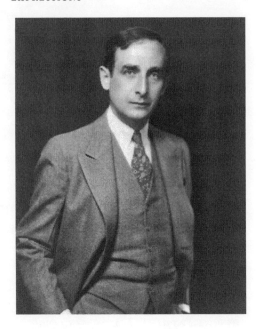

Harry Goldblatt

The initial impetus for Goldblatt's work was to mimic the microvascular arteriolar narrowings occurring in end-stage glomerulonephritis. Surprisingly, the clinical manifestations of macrovascular renal artery disease in humans had not been recognized at the time of his initial experimental studies.

Characterization of Renal Artery Occlusive Disease

Renal artery occlusive disease represents a collection of heterogeneic pathologic lesions. The histologic type and morphologic character of these stenoses are relevant to their clinical presentation and preferred treatment. The first comprehensive characterization of these diseases was proposed in the 1970s by Edgar G. Harrison, MD, and Lawrence McCormack, MD, two senior anatomic pathologists from the Mayo and Cleveland Clinics, respectively. Subsequently, the most widely used classification of renal artery disease, representing a modification of work from the former physicians, evolved from the University of Michi-

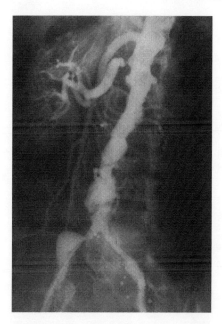

Arteriosclerotic renal artery
stenosis, representing aortic-
spillover disease

gan group. Included were arteriosclerotic, fribrodysplastic, and developmental stenoses

Arteriosclerotic stenoses are the most frequently encountered form of renal artery occlusive disease, accounting for 95% of all renal artery narrowings causing renovascular hypertension. Men are twice as likely as women to be affected with this disease. The mean age at the time of recognition for both genders has been approximately 55 years.

Two forms of renal artery arteriosclerosis exist, with overlaps occurring frequently. The first occurs as an arteriosclerotic plaque intrinsic to the renal artery, usually a half-centimeter beyond the aortic origin of the vessel. This type of renal artery arteriosclerosis is usually unilateral. The second form develops as an aortic plaque that spills over into the orifice of the renal artery. Nearly 80% of patients with renal artery arteriosclerosis and renovascular hypertension have aortic spillover disease. This form of renal artery arteriosclerosis is bilateral in 75% of cases. Intrarenal arteriosclerosis of second and third order branches occurs in less than 5% of these patients, being encountered most commonly in diabetic patients.

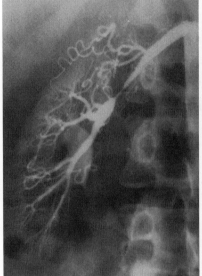
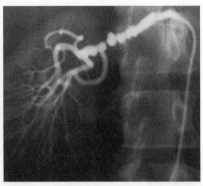
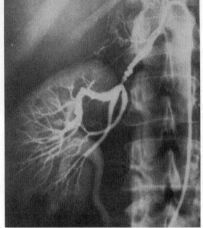

Arterial fibrodysplactic renal artery
stenoses: Intimal fibroplasia, Medial
fibrodysplasia, and Perimedial dysplasia

Fibrodysplastic stenoses may be categorized into lesions that affect
the intima, the media, or the perimedial-adventitial regions of the artery.

Intimal fibroplasia most often affects children, adolescents, or young
adults, with no known gender predilection. Intimal fibroplasia accounts
for approximately 5% of all fibrodysplastic renal artery lesions, with the
primary form of this disease usually being unilateral. It has the appearance of a solitary smooth circumferential narrowing, most often affecting the distal main renal artery.

Medial fibrodysplasia invariably affects women, predominantly during their childbearing years, with most patients presenting during their
fourth decade of life. These lesions account for approximately 85% of all
renal artery fibrodysplastic stenoses. Medial fibrodysplasia is most likely
to occur in the distal and middle thirds of the main renal artery with

approximately 25% of patients exhibiting extension into first-order renal artery branches. This disease has the appearance of a "string of beads." Bilateral disease exists in 60% of patients, but only 10% to 15% have functionally important disease of both renal arteries. The etiology of medial fibrodysplasia appears related to excessive physical forces on the renal artery associated with ptotic kidneys, and the effect that these physical forces have on the smooth muscle cells exposed to high estrogen levels causing them to enter into a secretory state, reflecting their transformation into myofibroblasts.

Perimedial dysplasia is the last of the fibrodysplastic diseases, accounting for approximately 10% of these lesions. This disease also occurs predominantly in women, presenting most often during the fifth decade of life. It has an appearance of serial stenoses without intervening mural aneurysms such as affect medial fibrodysplasia. Approximately 20% of patients with this type of lesion have bilateral disease, with extension into segmental vessels being very uncommon. This dysplastic disease frequently has coexistent renal artery segments manifesting medial fibrodysplasia.

Developmental stenoses represent another distinct category of renal artery occlusive disease. There is no gender predilection for this lesion. Its recognition occurs most often in children, at an average age of 10 years. All three elements of the vessel wall are abnormal with histologic evidence of secondary intimal fibroplasia, fragmentation of the internal elastic lamina, disruption of the media, and excess accumulation of elastic tissue in the perimedial-subadventitial tissues. Developmental

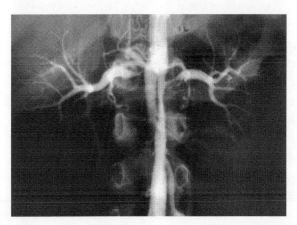

Developmental ostial renal artery stenoses associated with an abdominal aortic coarctation

lesions are frequently associated with abdominal aortic coarctations and often are encountered in patients with neurofibromatosis. Sixty-five percent of those patients having coexisting abdominal aortic coarctations have multiple renal arteries, suggesting that their disease evolves during embryonic times when the two dorsal aortae are fusing and the multiple metanephric vessels are disappearing.

Renin-Angiotensin System

Renin, when released in excess from the kidney's juxtaglomerular apparatus, initiates a sequence of events that contribute to high blood pressure. Renin is secreted following a number of stimuli, one of which is a pressure change accompanying renal artery occlusive disease that is sensed by the baroreceptors in the region of the mesangium of the glomerulus. Renin, a proteolytic enzyme, acts on the renin substrate angiotensinogen, an alpha-2 globulin produced in the liver, to form the dectapeptide angiotensin I. Converting enzyme subsequently cleaves two amino acids from angiotensin I to form angiotensin II. Angiotensin II is a profound arterial vasoconstrictor and provides the vasoactive element observed in renovascular hypertension. Furthermore, angiotensin II acts in a secondary fashion on the adrenal gland to enhance production of aldosterone, which facilitates sodium retention. The latter provides the volume element of renovascular hypertension.

Jean E. Sealey, DSc, performed classic studies that defined the role of renin release from the kidney into the systemic circulation. Her studies, performed nearly 25 years ago in New York City involving normotensive and essential hypertensive patients, confirmed that there is a constant release of renin from both kidneys, at levels 48% more than that noted in the peripheral circulation. If the total level of renal renin release exceeded 48%, its normal degradation appeared inadequate and hyper-reninemia with renin-mediated elevations of blood pressure occurs. In most individuals without renovascular hypertension, if the renin from an ischemic kidney increases, the opposite kidney's release of renin becomes suppressed, so that the sum of renin from both kidneys does not exceed 48% of that in the peripheral circulation. ·

Renal Artery Imaging

Simple anatomic existence of a renal artery stenosis is not an adequate predictor of its functional importance, unless associated with a pressure gradient sufficient enough to generate inappropriate renin release. Pressure gradients usually evolve only after a renal artery stenosis reaches an 80% level. Recognition of such critical lesions becomes important in clinical practice and may be evident by the arteriographic appearance of collateral vessels circumventing the narrowing. Joseph Bookstein, MD, at the University of Michigan, was one of the nation's leaders in establishing the functional importance of a hemodynamic stenosis when associated with collateral vessels.

D. Eugene Strandness, MD, at the University of Washington, is best known for his contributions to the development of duplex ultrasonography. He was one of the first to apply this technology to assessments of renovascular disease. Because of the two-dimensional aspects of ultrasonography, direct imaging may not always reveal a stenosis. Thus, velocity studies may prove more reliable for the identification of hemodynamic important renal artery stenoses. Such stenoses are usually associated with peak velocities in the range of 180 to 200 cm/sec and a ratio of these velocities to those in the aorta that approaches 3.5. Because it is difficult to discriminate among lesions exceeding 60% cross-sectional narrowing, as well as recognize small accessory or segmental vessel disease, this technology must be used cautiously as a means of excluding a diagnosis of renovascular hypertension. Needless to say the numerous tests available to document the relevance of renal artery disease confirm the inadequacy of existing studies, which in general have less than a 90% sensitivity and 80% specificity.

Surgical Techniques

Operative intervention should be carefully tailored for the specific renal artery disease being treated. A considerable number of surgical alternatives exist.

Endarterectomy has been the preferred method of many surgeons for the treatment of arteriosclerotic renal artery disease. Norman E.

Freeman, MD, an innovative surgeon, performed the first renal end-arterectomy for hypertension in 1952. He included among his students, Edwin J. (Jack) Wylie, MD. Wylie and Freeman subsequently practiced together for a brief period, and shortly thereafter, in 1951, Wylie performed the first aortoiliac endarterectomy in the United States. These procedures were the forerunners of the subsequent endarterectomy of the visceral branches of the aorta including the renal arteries. Wylie along with Ronald J. Stoney, MD, and others at the University of California, San Francisco popularized aortorenal endarterectomy for the treatment of renovascular hypertension.

Autogenous saphenous vein aortorenal bypass is today the most common surgical means of treating renovascular hypertension. This form of renal revascularization was first performed by Marion (Bill) DeWeese, MD, at the University of Michigan. The use of autogenous vein as a means of treating renovascular hypertension was subsequently popularized by William J. Fry, MD, Calvin B. Ernst, MD, and myself at the University of Michigan. Near-simultaneous publications were also forthcoming from John H. Foster, MD, and Richard H. Dean, MD, who also had an extensive experience with aortorenal vein graft procedures at Vanderbilt University.

Use of synthetic vascular prostheses for many renal artery reconstructions is acceptable, although such conduits may be difficult to use when anastomoses involve small vessels. Furthermore, they have an inherent predilection to develop luminal thrombus as well as anastomotic neointimal hyperplasia, and clearly they are much more subject to infection than autologous tissue grafts.

The surgical management of pediatric renovascular hypertension has been subject to recent changes. Because many vein grafts may become aneurysmal when used for aortorenal bypasses among pediatric patients, they should no longer be used in the treatment of children with renovascular hypertension. Free arterial grafts, usually with the hypogastric vessel, have been used for aortorenal bypasses for many age groups, and they are a particularly favored graft in children. The University of Michigan surgeons recently have advocated treating pediatric patients with orificial lesions by resection of the stenotic area, spatulation of the distal normal renal artery, and reimplantation of it into the aorta or into an adjacent renal artery if the lesion involves a segmental vessel. This technique has eliminated the risks attending late changes in autogenous vein and has facilitated the completion of relatively complex reconstructions in these young patients with a single anastomosis.

Nonanatomic renal artery reconstructions are frequently used to avoid hazards of directly clamping the aorta during conventional revascularizations. The utility of these procedures was established more than two decades ago by John A. Libertino, MD, and Andrew C. Novick, MD, from the Lahey Clinic and Cleveland Clinic, respectively. These forms of reconstructions, in particular, hepatorenal and splenorenal bypasses, have been preferred by many groups. Clearly, the celiac artery must not be diseased when using the splenic artery or hepatic artery as sites for origin of grafts.

Ex vivo renal artery reconstructions are appropriate in certain patients with complex disease, especially that affecting multiple segmental vessels associated with aneurysmal disease. This alternative therapy has been popularized most by surgeons responsible for major kidney transplantation programs, in particular Folkert O. Belzer, MD, and Johan L.Terpestra, MD, from the University of Wisconsin and Leiden University in the Netherlands, respectively.

Outcomes

The results of surgical therapy have been relatively consistent within the three specific subgroups of renal artery disease, namely, arteriosclerotic stenoses, fibrodysplastic stenoses, and developmental stenoses in the pediatric age group.

Benefits in treating arteriosclerotic renovascular hypertension are the least salutary among the various types of renal artery stenotic disease. Only 30% are cured and an additional 50% improved after a satisfactory renal revascularization. The remainder do not benefit from any surgical intervention. In these cases it is important to realize that upwards of 30% of patients presenting with this form of renal artery disease have underlying essential hypertension. In such cases removal of the renin-mediated component of their hypertension may be beneficial, but medical therapy must often continue for the treatment of their essential hypertension. The role of surgical therapy for renal artery occlusive disease in patients having ischemic nephropathy with renal failure is a subject of controversy. It would appear that this particular group of patients may benefit most, if indeed their renal function can be improved by a revascularization procedure.

Because essential hypertension is less likely in younger women with a fibrodysplastic renal artery narrowing, the benefits of surgical therapy are much better, with approximately 60% being cured and an additional 35% being improved after a technically successful surgical intervention. Because essential hypertension de facto does not exist in the pediatric age group, technically satisfactory reconstructive procedures are likely to eliminate the hypertensive state in nearly 80% of these children, with less than 5% not benefiting. Among all patients being treated for reno-vascular hypertension they experience the greatest benefit.

Contemporary surgical techniques provide considerable benefit to carefully selected patients with renovascular hypertension and should be considered the standard by which other therapeutic measures are assessed, such as percutaneous transluminal angioplasty. The best man-agement of the majority of patients with renal artery occlusive disease and renin-mediated hypertension continues to be surgical restoration of normal renal blood flow.

10

THE MICHIGAN LEGACY:
50 YEARS OF UNRAVELING THE RENAL ARTERY
AND SEVERE HYPERTENSION

This address was presented as the 24th Jobst Lecture at the University of Michigan on September 24, 2013, in Ann Arbor, Michigan. The Lecture, the Jobst Vascular Research Laboratories, and a Research Fellowship were established by Carolyn Jobst in honor of her husband, Conrad Jobst. The first Jobst Lecturer was given by Michael E. DeBakey in 1989. The current lecture affirms the important role the University of Michigan has played in defining the relevance of renal artery disease and renovascular hypertension.

The Michigan legacy of 50 years of unraveling the renal artery and severe hypertension is indeed a rich one. There have been many changes in our medical campus since 1963, when I was entering my senior year in medical school, to the present day, but the culture has not changed. It has been a very fertile one for discovery and care. The recognition that the kidney and perhaps the renal artery played important roles in high blood pressure were first recognized in 1898 by Robert Tigerstedt and Per Bergman, who identified a pressor substance found in the kidneys, which when injected intravenously cause a nearly 20 mmHg increase in the blood pressure. Nearly a half-century later in 1940 Irving Page and O.M.Helmer continued the refinement of these substances shortly after Eduardo Braun-Menendez had identified renin.

There have been many colleagues and mentors during the past half-century who have been instrumental in Michigan's contribution to understanding hypertensive diseases. Sibley W. Hoobler was one of the

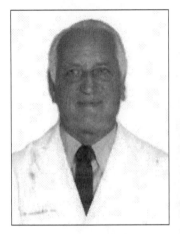

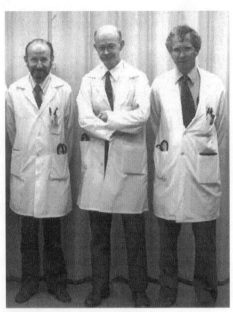

Sibley Hoobler (above)

Stevo Julius, David Bassett,
Andrew Zweifler (right)

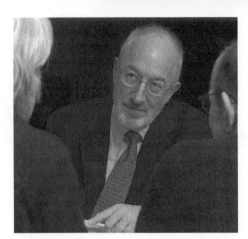

Alan Weder

most prominent of these leaders, who in 1946 established a Hypertension Division within the Department of Medicine, a group he headed
for nearly three decades. In 1957 he hosted a conference in Ann Arbor
attended by Irving Page from Cleveland as well as Eduardo Braun-
Menendez from Argentina, and it was during this meeting that the term
"angiotensin" was coined. The Hypertension Division had many stel-

lar faculty, including Andrew Zweifler, who was one of the institution's most outstanding teacher's and David Bassett, who was a lipid expert. Dr. Hoobler's successor was Stevo Julius, who became the Division Head in 1974, a position he held for the next 25 years. His legacy is clearly visible in *Adventures in Hypertension,* a memoir he authored that is indeed an exceptionally personal description of Michigan's role in defining the basis for hypertension. Alan Weder became the Head of the Hypertension Division in 1999, and was my partner in clinical practice for the last few decades. Alan is as complete a physician as anyone I have worked with since I joined the Michigan faculty in 1972.

The second investigator in the hypertension world who put Michigan on the map was Jerome W. Conn. He had attended the University of Michigan Medical School and was actually an intern in the Department of Surgery before switching to Internal Medicine. He served as the Head of the Endocrinology and Metabolism Division for three decades, retiring in 1974. Dr. Conn, best known in hypertensive circles for the recognition of primary aldosteronism, was a great supporter of the young. In his address to the Central Society he noted, "I am not old enough to have forgotten completely the perspective of younger colleagues. Their aspirations are pointed in your direction. Let us set for them a proper sample of kindness, friendliness, and common decency." One of my prized documents is a letter of thanks from Dr. Conn commenting on how grateful he was to see one of his students grow into a caring physician. This note came after I had subjected him to a limb-saving arterial bypass in the 1970s. He was a gem and a special mentor.

The third major player of the last half-century in the area of hypertensive vascular disease was David F. Bohr. David was a 1942 graduate of the University's Medical School and was an outstanding regulatory physiologist. Most of his investigative work focused on the reactivity of vascular smooth muscle. David was an outstanding investigator and it is of note that he wrote his last RO1-NIH grant at age 90. He had been well recognized by his colleagues, having been the president of the American Physiological Society in 1978. Perhaps he is best remembered by his trainees, two of them, Drs. Webb and Dominczak, who in a memorial noted that "Dr. Bohr inspired and mentored numerous scientists and students, and many remember him as an important role model. He was as kind, fair, and generous as he was brilliant." Therein resides a secret of

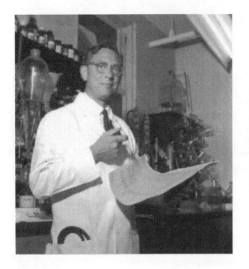
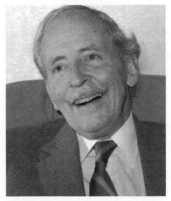

Jerome Conn (left) and
David Bohr (above)

Michigan's success at contributing new knowledge, namely helpful mentors and colleagues. David Bohr and Jerome Conn were outstanding examples of true professors and revered teachers.

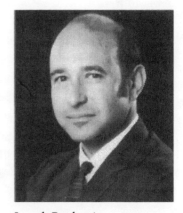

Two University of Michigan radiologists dominated the anatomic imaging of the renal artery in the 1970s. The first was Joseph Bookstein. He was an iconic interventional radiologist who recognized the relevance of collateral vessels as a means of documenting a hemodynamically significant as well as functionally significant renal artery lesion causing inappropriate renin release. He was creative and adventurous. At the same time John (Jack) R. Thornbury wrote extensively about the appropriate and inappropriate use of hypertensive urograms in the identification of renal artery and renin parenchymal diseases associated with hypertension. These two individuals were thoughtful and aggressive at pursuing conclusive diagnostic information regarding renovascular hypertension.

Joseph Bookstein

Although not often mentioned as an individual having much to do

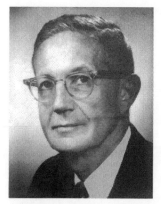

C Gardner Child

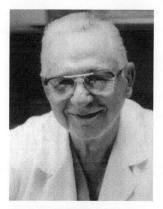

Marion (Bill) DeWeese

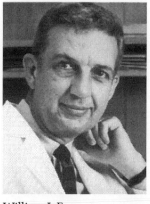

William J. Fry

with renovascular disease, C. Gardner Child had his beginnings very much grounded in that disease. Indeed, his first publication was a paper written with Irving Page on renovascular hypertension. He was the chairman of the Department of Surgery when I was a medical student and resident. Gardner was somewhat aristocratic, but he was one of my personal supporters, more so than any of the other senior faculty. He was the one who recruited me to the faculty after I finished my surgical residency. My sense is that he found joy in the success that a number of his trainees had as they pursued their academic interests in the field of hypertension.

Three other surgeons at Michigan also played a significant role in the past 50 years in the treatment of renovascular disease. The first was Marion (Bill) S. DeWeese, who made many original contributions to vascular surgery, perhaps the most important in his having performed the world's first aortorenal bypass in a human being. He also was the first to plicate the vena cava to prevent fatal pulmonary emboli, and he performed the first aortocoronary bypass in an animal model. From a personal perspective he was quite influential in my own life. I had been accepted to become a resident in the Internal Medicine program at the University of Michigan, but because of my experience on his service as an extern my senior year, I made a transition to the surgical training program. Two other individuals who were among my strongest mentors as a resident included William J. Fry, who

was one of the most intuitive surgeons I
have ever known, and Calvin B. Ernst.

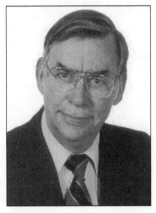

Cal Ernst became one of my closest
professional friends. He and I later became
co-editors of *The Journal of Vascular Surgery* even though we were at different institutions at the time. It's likely that our collaboration had evolved from our editing,
with Dr. Fry, a book *Renovascular Hypertension* that was published in 1984. At that
time no other monograph on the surgical
treatment of this disease existed.

Calvin B. Ernst

Another individual with Michigan roots
who was a close friend and mentor was
Ralph Straffon, who graduated from the University of Michigan's Medical School in 1953. Earlier he had been the captain of Michigan's football
team and was featured in a *Life* magazine article regarding his student
days. But his real talent came about after he finished a urology residency
at Michigan and assumed the role of the Chief of Urology at Cleveland
Clinic, then the Chief of Surgery, and then their Chief of Staff. Ralph
made many contributions in the area of renovascular disease and was
a valued critic of my younger career and the surgical activities in Ann
Arbor as they matured during the early 1970s.

There are two major issues regarding renal artery stenotic disease
related to hypertension. The first are the rheologic consequences that
may be defined by imaging, and the second are the hormonal consequences, which involve the renin angiotensin system. Perhaps one area
where the most original contributions had been made by the Michigan
faculty related to the former in defining the hemodynamic importance
of these stenoses. Clearly a gradient pressure in the 10 to 15 mmHg range
will allow the evolution of collaterals to circumvent the narrowed area
and that was a major focus of clinical research by Joseph Bookstein, who
undertook many studies involving the pharmacologic manipulation of
these vessels in the clinical arena to confirm their importance. Martin
R. Prince was a later addition to the Department of Radiology. In my
mind he is the father of magnetic resonant arteriographic evaluations
of renal artery disease. His contributions, including the development

of the breath-held technique of gadolinium imaging enhancement, has been a major contribution to our evaluating the hemodynamic importance of renal artery narrowings.

The hormonal or functional consequences of renal artery stenoses have been relatively well- understood with the knowledge that renin substrate, an alpha-2 globulin produced in the liver, is converted by the proteolytic enzyme, renin, to produce angiotensin I. This dectapeptide has little function but when acted up by converting enzyme forms angiotensin II, an octapeptide, which is a profound vasoconstrictor that indirectly acts on the adrenal gland to increase aldosterone production with the subsequent retention of sodium and water molecules. Thus the release of renin in excessive amounts has both vasoconstrictive and volume elements.

The relationship of these agents to known renal artery disease was the focus of studies by Jean Sealey in New York City, who noted that in nonrenovascular patients the amount of renin coming from each kidney was usually 24% more than entered the kidney. This recognition had been developed further by E. Darracott Vaughan who was working in Sealey's lab. He noted that patients who were cured of renovascular hypertension all had an excess of renin release being greater than 48% more than entered the ischemic kidney compared to the evidence of nonhypersecretion when the patient did not benefit from treatment of a unilateral renal artery narrowing. In 1975 our laboratory published similar data looking at individual kidney production of renin and documented the prognostic value of using the renal: systemic renin indices to define those patients who might be cured or those who might be improved after a unilateral renal artery reconstruction. This work provided a benchmark that stood the test of time. However, renin profiling is uncommon in contemporary practice because of the intense patient preparation and catheterizations required.

The importance of the renin-angiotensin system in hypertension and its contribution to accelerating significant nonrenal vascular diseases, including coronary artery and carotid disease, has clearly been established. Interestingly both the genes for renin and angiotensinogen exist on chromosome 1 and actually are present in multicellular animals having no circulation. The fact is that angiotensin II is a significant inflammatory mediator that is likely to contribute to plaque instability and progression, both of which contribute to accelerated atherosclerotic vascular disease. That means that elevated blood pressures due to renovascular disease may be more life-threatening than when occurring as part of essential hypertension.

The University of Michigan has had a broad experience in the surgical management of arteriosclerotic renovascular hypertension. Our group was one of the first to note a difference in surgical outcomes of bypass procedures taken for arteriosclerosis isolated to the renal artery in comparison to the less salutary outcomes when the same lesion was associated with nonrenal artery atherosclerosis affecting the carotid, coronary, or extremity arteries. The treatment, being a bypass or an endarterectomy and in more recent times percutaneous transluminal angioplasty (PTA) with stenting, may all be appropriate interventions in properly selected patients. However, the treatment algorithm is quite complex, and the specific management of these patients requires an understanding of this complexity. Nonanatomic reconstructions because of a hostile aorta or cardiac compromise are appropriate in select patients.

The first report of balloon angioplasty of an atherosclerotic renal artery lesion was Andreas Grüntzig's *Lancet* paper in 1974. More recently a number of prospective randomized studies comparing PTA to medical treatment of atherosclerotic renal artery disease have concluded that catheter-based interventions have no value over drug treatment. However, all these studies to date have been highly criticized, and at least from my own personal perspective the selection of patients for none of these investigations was done with the same rigor that had been done at the University of Michigan when selecting patients for a bypass or an endarterectomy.

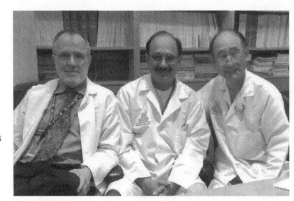

David Williams, Nara
Dasika, Kyung Cho

The fact of the matter is that for over a quarter of a century the University of Michigan has had three outstanding clinical radiologists who have superb judgment and simply extraordinary technical expertise catheter-based interventions. David M. Williams, Nara Dasika, and Kyung J. Cho have provided images and catheter-skills unequalled by their peers throughout the nation.

Arterial fibrodysplasia, the second most common cause of renovascular hypertension, was first subcategorized at the University of Michigan into intimal fibroplasia, medial fibroplasia, and perimedial dysplasia. A classic paper on the histopathologic character and current etiologic concepts was published by our group in 1975 and has continued to be the benchmark regarding this topic. The ultrastructure of arterial fibroplasia was further defined by Vikrom Sottiurai, who was an anatomy instructor and a resident in our surgical training program at the same time. The electron microscopy of both medial fibrodysplasia and perimedial dysplasia that he had described remain the classic description of this disease at a more subcellular level.

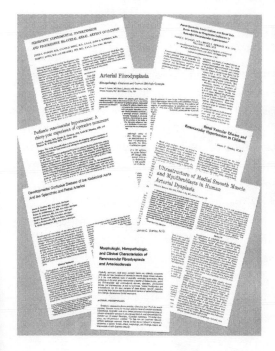

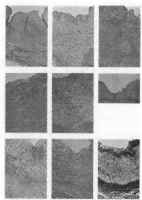

FMD publications and histology.

The treatment of fibrodysplastic renal artery diseases causing reno-vascular hypertension is also complex. However, the appropriateness of PTA as a first means of therapy has been established when there is no disease involving the segmental vessels or true aneurysms involving major branchings of the diseased artery. The University of Michigan has contributed significantly to the understanding of reconstructive surgery using autogenous saphenous vein in the form of aortorenal bypasses and has published widely on the technology, including spatulation of the anastomoses and follow-up to assess the adequacy of the recon-struction for years following the initial procedure.

The third type of renal artery disease that has been recognized to be an exceedingly important cause of hypertension relates to the devel-opmental stenoses. The initial University of Michigan experience was associated with many patients who had neurofibromatosis-1. In part these individuals came from a large pool of children who had been fol-lowed by John F. Holt, who was the head of our Pediatric Radiology group and who had an interest in the musculoskeletal aspects of neu-rofibromatosis-1. A small number of these patients were found to have refractory hypertension and as imaging became available were found to have ostial narrowings of their renal artery with relatively normal vas-cular architecture elsewhere.

The favored treatment for these lesions has been aortic reimplanta-tion of the more normal renal artery, which has been transected beyond the stenosis. This management protocol is less complex that a bypass. However, some lesions that affected the more distal renal artery are best treated with a bypass using a hypogastric artery free graft. Our group was the first to report the late consequences of using autogenous saphenous vein in children, which regardless of how carefully it was handled and prepared became aneurysmal as a likely consequence of mural ischemia with inadequate function of vasa vasorum in the veins of the young.

A related issue regarding the renin angiotensin system and renal artery disease is a subgroup of patients who had midabdominal coarc-tations. Many of these individuals had multiple renal arteries and, like those with renal artery disease, neurofibromatosis was evident in more than 20% of the patients. The reconstruction of these individuals was quite complex. In 2006 our group reported the largest series of these individuals, numbering over 50, all of whom had successful surgical

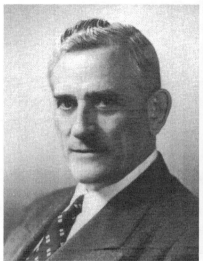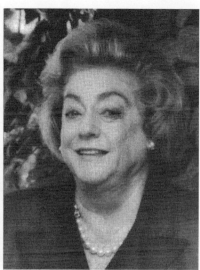

Conrad and Caroline Jobst

outcomes. Many of these individuals required concomitant renal or splanchnic artery reconstructions in addition to their aortic repairs.

Any discussion of Michigan's legacy regarding the renal artery and renovascular hypertension must include a comment about renal artery aneurysms. In 1995 we reported our experience with over 252 aneurysms in 168 patients, which represented the largest experience with this disease ever published. A small percentage of these individuals had associated renin-mediated hypertension as a consequence of the aneurysm either compressing or torqueing an adjacent renal artery. The risk of rupture of smaller aneurysms was exceedingly small and was not considered a justifiable reason to intervene either with an open operation or a catheter-based obliteration. A more aggressive approach seemed appropriate if secondary hypertension was a suspected result of the aneurysmal disease.

So how can I conclude my story about the journey that I have taken to witness this Michigan Legacy. Many thanks are due.

First, my deepest gratitude is owed to Caroline Jobst for founding this lectureship in honor of her husband, Conrad; for creating the Jobst fellowship; and for establishing the Conrad Jobst Vascular Laboratories.

Her gift has had a major impact on improving our understanding of vascular disease.

Second, a busy academic life is a team effort, and I owe thanks to the more than a hundred individuals who have authored abstracts and papers with me on renal artery disease and renovascular hypertension during the past three decades. Included among these authors are many of our 33 vascular surgery fellows and residents having trained here since the program was first initiated in 1974. And of course many contributions to this Michigan Legacy have come from the 23 vascular surgery faculty I have worked with since 1972. *(All of these individuals are identified in the appended lists at the conclusion of this address).*

Lastly, I am very grateful to those patients with renal artery disease who entrusted their lives to my care. There were many memorable individuals from distant continents, arriving after traveling thousands of miles to meet a team of strangers to care for them, including the young, who are completely helpless, and the older, some of whom were very sophisticated in their expectations of getting the best care. The Michigan faculty and staff did not let them down, and that is our legacy.

Let me remind you that a legacy is a gift we pass on to those who follow us. It is not a reputation laid out on a document or an ego badge. It's really what we give. Considering the many at Michigan who have given to our understanding and betterment of care for those with renal artery disease and secondary hypertension, I would say that the Michigan Legacy regarding renovascular hypertension is a very secure gift to the future of medicine.

THE TEAM MEMBERS

Coauthors of Abstracts and Papers on Renovascular Diseases

P.H. Abrahame, F. Afshinnia, G. Ailawadi, D.A. Axelrod, D.C. Barnhart, B.F. Bates, K.H. Berecek, R. Berguer, N.B. Blatt, M. Bitzer, D.F. Bohr, J.J. Bookstein, E.L. Bove, C.A. Braak, P.B. Brophy, J.D. Cardneau, R.C. Carlos, P.K. Castelli, C.Y. Chang, R.E. Cilley, K. Cho, E.L. Cohen, D.M. Coleman, A.C. Coran, J.A. Cowan, E. Criado, J.L. Cronenwett, N.L. Dasika, J.R. Dillman, J.B. Dimick, Q. Dong, F.E. Eckhauser, J.L. Eliason, E.E. Erlandson, C.B. Ernst, A.M. Fendrick, C.P. Fischer, D.P. Flanigan, J.B. Froehlich, W.J. Fry, D.G. .Fryback, B.L. Gewertz, L.M. Graham, V. Grigoryants, C.E. Grim, L.J. Greenfield, P.K. Henke, G.L. Hoffman, M.J. Horan, L.A. Jacobs, A. Kazmers, D.B. Kershaw, B.S. Knipp, J.W. Konnak, R.J. Lederman, S.M. Lindenauer, F.J. Londy, F.F. Marshall, L.M. Messina, J.F.M. Meaney, J.G. Modrall, M. Nanamori, T.T. Nostrant, R.R. Neubig, R.G. Ohye, J.F. Porush, M.R. Prince, M.S. Proctor, S.B. Proctor, P. Rao, J.E. Rectenwald, E.J. Rocella, E.L. Rhodes, J. Sadushima, R.H. Samson, R. Sarkar, A.A. Sharathkumar, E.A. Smith, T.A. Sos, V.S. Sottiurai, V.L. Street, B. Sundaram, J.M. Terris, J.P. Tullis, J.R. Thornbury, G.R. Upchurch Jr, R. Vellody, G. Vidt, T.W. Wakefield, J.F. Walter, J.S. Ward, N.C. Watson, A.B. Weder, T.H. Welling III, W.M. Whitehouse Jr, D.M. Williams, K.A. Yao, and G.B. Zelenock

Vascular Surgery Trainees

Andris Kazmers, Thomas Wakefield, Timothy Kresowik, Thomas Brothers, Rachel Podrazik, Thomas Whitehill, Thomas Huber, Mohammad Moursi, Charles Shanley, Keith Ozaki, Gregory Modrall, Rajabrata Sarkar, Peter Henke, Joseph Downing, Matthew Eagleton,

Steven Posner, Jonathan Eliason, John Rectenwald, Christopher Longo, Matthew Campbell, Loay Kabbani, Guillermo Escobar, Justin Hurie, Dawn Coleman, Shipra Arya, Frank Vandy, Nicholas Osborne, Paul Dimusto, Jordan Knepper, Danielle Campbell, Tina Chen, Danielle Horne, Anna Eliassen

Vascular Surgery Faculty Partners

William Fry, Calvin Ernst, S. Martin Lindenauer, William Gross, Gerald Zelenock, Jack Cronenwett, Walter Whitehouse Jr, Errol Erlandson, Thomas Wakefield, Louis Messina, Linda Graham, Charles Shanley, Gilbert Upchurch Jr, Peter Henke, Matthew Eagleton, Sunita Srivastava, John Rectenwald, Ramon Berguer, Enrique Criado, Jonathan Eliason, Guillermo Escobar, Katherine Gallagher, Dawn Coleman

VASCULAR SURGERY

The first two of these three addresses are summaries of clinical practices, which at the time of their presentation represented the largest reported experiences with pediatric renovascular hypertension and abdominal aortic coarctations, respectively. The third address is a review of visceral artery aneurysms, in particular those affecting the splanchnic and renal arteries. Little philosophy can be found in these addresses, but they represent an accurate accounting of the Michigan Difference in caring for patients with very unique vascular diseases.

11

PEDIATRIC RENOVASCULAR HYPERTENSION: CONTEMPORARY SURGICAL TREATMENT

This work was presented at the 60th Annual Meeting of the Society for Vascular Surgery on June 1, 2006, in Philadelphia, Pennsylvania. It was subsequently published in an expanded form in J Vasc Surg 44:1219–29, 2006.

Renal artery occlusive disease affecting pediatric-aged patients is an important, but very uncommon cause of childhood hypertension. Pediatric renovascular hypertension when unrecognized and untreated has been associated with serious complications including hemorrhagic stroke, hypertensive encephalopathy with impaired mental development, and failure to thrive. Poorly controlled hypertension may result in left ventricular hypertrophy and severe diastolic dysfunction. Additionally, when the entire renal mass is involved, flash pulmonary edema associated with renal insufficiency may occur.

Pediatric renal artery stenoses represent a spectrum of heterogeneous diseases, although developmental anomalies, often with concomitant narrowings of the splanchnic arteries and the abdominal aorta, are most common. The impetus for the present report was to document the University of Michigan experience, which is the largest reported encounter with this disease, and in more contemporary times has included exceedingly complicated lesions requiring complex surgical interventions.

Patients and Clinical Manifestations. From 1963 to 2006, 97 children with sustained hypertension caused by renal artery occlusive disease underwent operation at the University of Michigan Medical Center

(University Hospital and Mott Children's Hospital). Fifty-seven of these patients were the subject of three prior reports, each reflecting different eras of management. The more contemporary era encompassed 40 patients treated from 1994 to 2006. The profile of these patients was unusual in that those groups where an inflammatory aortoarteritis might be suspect were in a distinct minority. Three children were Asian, four were Hispanic, two were African-American, and the remaining 88 were Caucasian.

The children's gender and pattern of renal and nonrenal disease was revealing. Patients ranged in age from three months to 17 years. The series included 58 boys and 39 girls whose mean ages were 8.8 and 11.4 years, respectively. The mean age of the entire group of children was 9.8 years. Gender differences were even more notable in the 21 boys and 11 girls who had coexistent aortic disease. Follow-up ranged from 3 months to 42 years, and averaged 4.2 years.

Blood Pressure Status. The mean duration of known preoperative hypertension was 10.5 months. The mean preoperative blood pressure before drug treatment was 178/105 mmHg, and 155/94 mmHg with drug therapy. All but one of the 97 patients had poor control of hypertension at the time of surgical treatment. Blood pressures were categorized using the most updated reports of expected pediatric blood pressures based on age and gender.

Patients were classified as *cured* if for the preceding six months they were taking no antihypertensive medications and they were normotensive, defined as blood pressures below the expected 95th percentile. Patients were considered *improved* if their blood pressures were within normotensive ranges while on drug therapy exclusive of angiotensin converting enzyme (ACE) inhibitors, or if their diastolic pressures were greater than normal but 15% lower than preoperative levels. Patients were considered therapeutic *failures* when their diastolic pressures were greater than the normal levels and not 15% lower than preoperative levels or ACE inhibitors were required for blood pressure control.

Asymptomatic hypertension was common in the series' adolescent patients. Nevertheless, nearly half the older patients had left ventricular hypertrophy reflecting long-standing hypertension. Fatigue, lethargy, and cephalalgia were noted in some of the older children. In contrast, symptomatic hypertension and failure to thrive was often present in the very young. Six of this series' younger patients had hypertensive seizures, including three who had strokes as the initial manifestation of their hypertension. Only one patient, the series youngest, had severe deterioration of renal function due to occlusion of both renal arteries. He presented with multiple episodes of flash-pulmonary edema requiring intubation prior to his transfer to the authors' institution Two additional patients had moderate renal insufficiency with distinct evidence of nephrosclerosis of the kidney opposite the one affected with the renal artery stenosis.

Renal Artery Disease. Complex medial and perimedial dysplastic disease, complicated with secondary intimal fibroplasia, accounted for all but a few of the renal artery stenoses in this series. Only four patients had clear evidence of an inflammatory arteritis, including the series' only documented case of Takayasu's disease and two patients with Moyamoya disease. Unilateral stenoses affected 65 patients and bilateral stenoses were evident in the 32 remaining children. Among those patients with bilateral disease, six presented initially with unilateral disease, with contralateral renal artery narrowings evolving distant from their first recognized disease.

Ostial stenoses affected all 35 patients having abdominal aortic narrowings and 34 of the 62 patients exhibiting no aortic pathology. These arteries often had a gross hourglass appearance with visible narrowings immediately adjacent to the aorta. However, the most critical narrowing was often within the aortic wall itself and not grossly visible, being recognized only on arteriographic studies. Ostial narrowings, considered developmental in etiology, occurred most often among this series' 23 patients having evidence of neurofibromatosis-1 (NF-1). Midrenal arterial stenoses were encountered less frequently in this updated experience, affecting only three of the most recently treated 40 patients, whereas 12 of 57 patients in our previously reported series exhibited midrenal lesions.

Extraparenchymal segmental renal artery stenoses affected 18 children as isolated lesions in 13 and in association with main renal artery disease in five children. Web-type second-order segmental stenoses in two patients were the only intraparenchymal lesions encountered in the series. Eight patients exhibited renal artery aneurysms. Five aneurysms occurred at renal artery bifurcations, and three affected the main renal artery, including one that appeared to be a post-stenotic aneurysm.

Concomitant Aortic and Splanchnic Arterial Disease. Abdominal aortic coarctations or hypoplasia affected 32 patients, including 19 who also had coexisting celiac artery or superior mesenteric artery ostial stenoses. Five additional children without aortic disease exhibited celiac and superior mesenteric arterial stenoses. Only two of the 24 patients with splanchnic artery lesions manifested classic intestinal angina. No patient with aortic or splanchnic arterial disease exhibited evidence of an acute inflammatory aortitis. Focal suprarenal abdominal aortic coarctations affected 12 patients, intrarenal coarctations affected 15 children, tubular infrarenal coarctations affected three children, a terminal aortic occlusion affected one child, and diffuse aortic hypoplasia extending from the celiac artery to the aortic bifurcation occurred in one patient. Multiple renal arteries were present in 82% of those children having abdominal aortic narrowings in close proximity to their renal arteries.

Diagnostic Assessment. Conventional, catheter-based arteriographic studies were undertaken in all but six patients. Most arteriograms involved a femoral artery approach. Abdominal aortography, with anteroposterior and lateral projections, was performed prior to selective catheterization of the renal and splanchnic arteries. Magnification renal arteriograms were obtained in oblique projections to assess segmental renal artery stenoses. Transaortic pressure measurements were used to determine pressure gradients across aortic narrowings when present.

Intravenous digital subtraction arteriography (IV DSA) has been used in small infants, with injection of contrast medium into the right atrium, followed by subtraction imaging. Thin-slice computed tomographic arteriography (CTA) has recently been used as a less invasive means of assessing the renal circulation. However, the large dose of radiation accompanying CTA make it less desirable. Magnetic resonance angiography (MRA) was often utilized to screen patients in this series, but because of frequent false positive studies, it has not been considered reliable enough to establish the exact degree of a renal artery stenosis.

Hypertensive urography was found in our early experience to be of limited value at establishing the presence of pediatric renovascular disease because of its lack of sensitivity to detect bilateral or segmental renal artery disease. In fact, no children in the last 25 years have had urograms used as a primary diagnostic test. Similarly, although abnormal renin production, reflected in elevated renal vein ratios or indices, has been well-documented in past University of Michigan reports, it was used only twice during the past decade in two patients with disease of equivocal importance. Abdominal duplex ultrasonography had value in following patients postoperatively, but was infrequently used as a primary diagnostic test.

Operative Therapy. Arterial reconstructive surgery for pediatric renovascular hypertension was individualized, taking into account the patient's anatomic renal artery disease, as well as splanchnic arterial and aortic disease. The author's experience included certain general tenets. First, use of a supraumbilical transverse abdominal incision was favored, with medial reflection of the viscera to allow wide exposure of the renal vasculature. Second, patients were systemically anticoagulated prior to aortic and renal artery clamping with the intravenous administration of sodium heparin, 150 units/kg. Third, at the conclusion of the arterial reconstruction, heparin anticoagulation was usually reversed with slow intravenous administration of protamine sulfate, 1.5 mg/100 units of previously administered heparin. Fourth, patients undergoing very small vessel reconstructions invariably were given aspirin intraoperatively through their nasogastric tube, to lessen the risk of platelet accumulation and thrombus formation at anastomotic sites. Fifth, maintenance of a diuresis at the time of renal artery dissection and reconstruction was facilitated by the intravenous administration of Mannitol, 0.17 grams/kg. Sixth, *in situ* reconstructions were preferred so as to not disrupt pre-existing collateral vessels. Only one *ex vivo* repair was undertaken in this series. Lastly, although staged procedures were common in the earlier University of Michigan experience, single-staged corrective operations have recently become standard practice.

Primary Renal Artery Surgery. A variety of surgical procedures have been undertaken. Bilateral procedures occurred 34 times, but accounted for only one of 20 procedures undertaken during the first decade of this experience, compared to 19 of the 40 most recently performed procedures. The most common surgical procedure was renal artery implantation into the aorta (n49), the main or segmental renal artery (n7), or the superior mesenteric artery (n3). Aortorenal bypasses with vein grafts were standard during the first decade of this experience (n25), but have not been favored during the past 25 years (n1). Instead, the internal iliac artery used as a free graft (n11) has become preferred for aortorenal bypasses. Iliorenal bypasses using vein grafts, usually covered with a Dacron mesh, have been performed when other forms of reconstructive procedures were not possible (n3). Splenorenal constructions with a direct anastomosis of the involved vessels (n2) were performed in the distant past, but are not favored in contemporary times because of coexistent or later development of a celiac artery stenosis. Resections of the stenotic renal artery with primary reanastomoses (n4), focal arterioplasties (n10), or open operative dilations (n4) were less common reconstructive procedures undertaken in this series. Primary nephrectomy was performed often for irreparable renal disease (n12) and infrequently (n1) for an unplanned technical failure of an intended vascular repair. The two most common primary operations: renal artery implantation and aortorenal bypass, deserve further comment.

Renal Artery Implantation. Implantation of the normal renal artery beyond an ostial stenosis into the aorta has become an important means of pediatric renal revascularization at the University of Michigan. In these circumstances, the transected renal artery is spatulated anteriorly and posteriorly, so as to create a generous anastomotic orifice. An oval aortotomy is made with an aortic punch, being a little more than twice the diameter of the renal artery being implanted. This provides a sufficiently large anastomosis, so as the child grows an anastomotic narrowing would not evolve. These anastomoses were usually performed using interrupted monofilament sutures. However, a continuous suture was often used in older adolescents with large renal arteries. Most implantations of the renal artery were into a normal infrarenal segment of the aorta. Medial mobilization of the kidney was often necessary to ensure that there was no tension on the implanted renal artery.

Implantation of a renal artery branch or accessory renal artery into a nondiseased adjacent main or segmental renal artery also involved spatulation of the segmental vessel and completion of the anastomo-

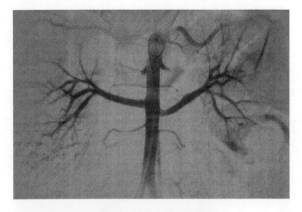

Reimplantation of
the renal artery into
the aorta

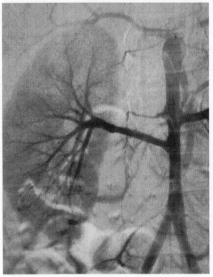

Aortorenal bypass with an internal iliac artery segment

sis using monofilament sutures. Implantation of a renal artery into the proximal superior mesenteric artery was undertaken when implantation elsewhere was deemed hazardous.

Aortorenal Bypass. The internal iliac artery is favored for pediatric renal bypasses. The excised internal iliac artery usually included its inferior branches, which are incised to create a large common orifice for the aortic anastomosis. Distal renal artery-to-graft anastomoses are completed following spatulation of both the iliac artery and renal artery, so as to increase the anastomotic circumference. Such ovoid anastomoses are less likely to develop late strictures, and in very young children are completed with interrupted sutures, although a continuous suture may be used in reconstructing larger renal arteries. Two patients with stenoses of multiple renal arteries required approximation of these vessels to each other to form a common orifice to which an aortorenal graft was then anastomosed.

Synthetic prosthetic grafts were not used for any of this series' primary renal artery procedures because of their potential infectivity, technical difficulties in anastomosing them to small arteries, and unpredictable long-term durability considering the many decades of life expectancy of these children. Similarly, vein grafts were noted to have a propensity to undergo late aneurysmal dilations, and because of this they are currently not used except when other forms of renal revascularization are impossible. When autogenous saphenous veins are used, a Dacron mesh is placed about the implanted vein.

Secondary Renal Artery Surgery. Nineteen patients underwent repeat renal procedures, when the primary revascularization proved unsuccessful. Nine secondary nephrectomies followed a failed or failing primary reconstructive procedure. No one primary procedure appeared more responsible for these reoperations, except for use of vein grafts with two children exhibiting microembolization of thrombi arising within their aneurysmal vein graft. Fifteen children underwent one reoperation, two underwent two secondary operations, and two others underwent three reoperations.

Aortic and Splanchnic Arterial Surgery. Aortic and splanchnic arterial reconstructions were performed at the time of renal artery operations in 25 and 15 patients, respectively, and at times distant from their renal procedures in an additional five and two patients, respectively. The specifics of these nonrenal operations deserve mention.

Patch Aortoplasty. Primary aortoplasty using a polytetrafluoroethylene (PTFE) patch (n18) has become the preferred means of treating isolated abdominal aortic coarctation or hypoplasia in children (Figure 7). Dacron patch aortoplasty (n1) utilized once in the early experience is no longer used because of the concern that this material may undergo late aneurysmal deterioration. Fifteen of these 19 patches were placed at the time of the renal operation. Patches were made sufficiently large enough so as to be least constrictive as the child grows into adulthood.

Thoracoabdominal Bypass. In certain instances a primary thoracoabdominal bypass was favored over an aortoplasty because of the patient's age and anatomic disease affecting the renal or splanchnic arteries. Fabricated Dacron prostheses (n3) were used in the early experience, but PTFE prostheses (n8) have been favored more recently. Extraperitoneal reflection of the abdominal viscera in these cases provided excellent access to the upper abdominal aorta when that was to be the site of the bypass origin. If a higher site was needed, a thoracotomy was performed and the graft was anastomosed to the supradiaphragmatic aorta. Grafts originating in the chest were easily tunneled through the posterior diaphragm, behind the left kidney to the distal aorta.

Splanchnic Arterial Reconstruction. Seventeen patients with developmental aortic and renal artery narrowings had critical ostial stenoses of their celiac and superior mesenteric arteries. In 15 patients, it proved advantageous to undertake reconstruction of these splanchnic arteries when treating their renovascular disease. The basis for this approach related in part to the potential difficulty of any future splanchnic vascular operation that might be needed, and the facility with which such could be accomplished at the same time of the renal revascularization. In five patients the normal celiac artery, after being transected beyond its ostial narrowing, was placed as a patch over the narrowed aortic origin of the superior mesenteric artery. In an additional five patients the mobilized superior mesenteric artery was directly implanted into the anterior aorta below the left renal vein.

Trends in the operative treatment of pediatric renovascular hypertension became apparent among the 132 primary renal operations of the current series. The 58 procedures performed during the last 12 years represented a much greater degree of complexity than undertaken in earlier years. The more recent operative experience substantiated the efficacy of renal artery implantations into the aorta, as well as single-staged reconstructions of coexisting abdominal aortic narrowings and splanchnic arterial stenoses.

Surgical Outcomes. The numbers of patients in any category of specific operative intervention were too small to justify life-table outcome analyses. Nevertheless, the salutary effects of operation on blood pressure control appear to justify surgical therapy. The mean blood pressure of all patients at the latest time of follow-up was 115/72 mmHg. Benefits regarding blood pressure control have accrued to 97% of children in the University of Michigan series following operative therapy. Hypertension was cured in 68 children (70%), improved in 26 (27%), and unchanged in three patients (3%). Long-term benefits were more common in the earlier experience.

Renal revascularization eliminated the recurrent episodes of progressive azotemia and flash pulmonary edema in the series' one patient with severe preoperative renal insufficiency. The combined number of primary and secondary nephrectomies reflected unreconstructable renal artery disease in more than half the cases. A potential worsening of renal function among those undergoing nephrectomy did not become a reality. In fact, despite the loss of renal mass, dialysis did not occur in any of the series' patients. There were no operative deaths. One late death due to a myocardial infarction occurred four years postoperatively in a patient with Takayasu's aortitis.

The optimal treatment of pediatric renovascular hypertension must be individualized given the child's specific renal artery disease. The University of Michigan experience with aortic implantation of renal arteries has been unique and avoids certain shortcomings of other procedures. Splenorenal reconstructions are rarely undertaken in contemporary practice, in that celiac artery ostial narrowings may evolve later as the child grows and result in recurrent hypertension. In addition, the use of autogenous vein should be avoided, given the experience that carefully prepared veins often underwent late aneurysmal deterioration. The logic of undertaking single-staged vascular reconstructive procedures when treating renal artery disease in concert with aortic or splanchnic arterial disease, receives support from the current experience. The alternative, a later operation in the same anatomic area to treat a second stenotic lesion, entails well-recognized difficulties and hazards of reoperations.

The appropriateness of undertaking surgical therapy in very small infants is ill-defined. Technical challenges exist in reconstructing renal arteries less than 2 mm in diameter and renal revascularization in these circumstances should be pursued only when uncontrolled severe hypertension or renal failure threaten the patient. Such was the case with the youngest University of Michigan patient who weighed only 4.7 kg at the time of operation for bilateral renal artery occlusions. Renal revascularizations are most likely to be successful after age two years and deferring reconstructive procedures in younger children when possible is reasonable. However, drug treatment of hypertension in the very young child may be difficult and requires frequent and fastidious monitoring.

The role of percutaneous transluminal angioplasty (PTA) in treating pediatric renovascular hypertension remains controversial. Failure following PTA for developmental disease might be anticipated, given the excessive elastic tissue in many stenoses that would predictably contribute to early postdilation recoil, as well as the minute caliber of these diseased vessels that might lead to their disruption when dilated. Nevertheless, a small number of recent reports suggest success with catheter-based interventions. It is of note that if the disease being treated is a quiescent inflammatory aortoarteritis, then more salutary outcomes would follow PTA than might be the case if treating developmentally hypoplastic renal arteries. However, even in the former setting recurrent stenoses are frequent.

In the very early University of Michigan experience, attempted PTA for orificial stenoses proved unsuccessful, and thereafter it was rarely pursued as a primary therapeutic modality. This caution was reinforced in that six of the series' most recently treated 40 patients were failures of PTA performed elsewhere prior to their being treated at the authors' institution. Nevertheless, catheter-based interventions were undertaken on two occasions in the University of Michigan experience. In the first patient an intraparenchymal stenosis affecting a second-order segmental branch not amenable to direct reconstruction was successfully treated by infusing alcohol into the diseased vessel with infarction of the distal renin-producing renal parenchyma. The second child had a focal web-like stenosis of a third-order segmental branch successfully dilated by PTA.

Pediatric renovascular hypertension is likely to be considered more frequently as children are screened for blood pressure and cardiac abnormalities more often. In the future less invasive diagnostic testing will facilitate confirmation of renal artery disease. Conventional surgical revascularization emphasizing direct renal artery implantations and single-staged concomitant aortic and splanchnic arterial reconstructions offers excellent results. However, these are challenging interventions, and the optimal care of these children requires carefully planned and deftly performed operations. Under such circumstances, more than 95% of these children should benefit from open surgical reconstructions.

12

ABDOMINAL AORTIC COARCTATION: SURGICAL THERAPY BY THORACOABDOMINAL BYPASS, PATCH AORTOPLASTY, AND INTERPOSITION AORTOAORTIC GRAFT

This work was presented at the 31ˢᵗ Annual Meeting of the Midwestern Vascular Surgical Society on September 7, 2007, in Chicago, Illinois. It was subsequently published in expanded form in J Vasc Surg 48:1073–82, 2008.

Coarctation of the abdominal aorta is a rare disease encompassing many differing etiologies and diverse methods of treatment The impetus for this presentation, which represents the largest reported experience involving patients with this disease, was to better define the anatomic and clinical character of this entity, as well as the technical issues and the adequacy of conventional open vascular reconstructive procedures in its treatment.

Patient Characteristics. Fifty-three patients with abdominal aortic coarctation underwent operative treatment at the University of Michigan Medical Center from 1963 to 2008. Forty-one of the series' patients have been treated since 1994. The series includes 34 male and 19 female patients, ranging in age from 2 to 49 years, with a mean age of 11.9 years. Patient ages, in years, were: 2–4 (n4), 5–8 (n17), 9–14 (n16), 15–20 (n11) and 25–49 (n5). Male patients outnumbered females 24:13 under age 15 years and 10:6 when 15 years or older.

Etiology. Developmental coarctations were suspected in the majority (n48) of this series' patients. A developmental etiology received support in the confirmed coexistence of neurofibromatosis-1 (NF-1) in 14 patients, an excessive number of multiple renal arteries in 16 of the 37 patients with suprarenal narrowings, Williams syndrome in one patient, and Alagille syndrome in another patient. Certain of the aortic narrowings exhibited atypical abdominal aortic coarctations having the characteristics of an inflammatory aortitis (n4). Balloon angioplasty of a thoracic aortic coarctation in a newborn at another hospital, complicated by aortic thrombosis, was considered the cause of an intrarenal coarctation (n1) in the series' remaining patient.

Aortic Disease. Extensive preoperative imaging of the aorta was undertaken in all patients. Imaging during the earlier years of this experience involved catheter-based aortography. MRA subsequently became a common diagnostic test, but conventional arteriography was often necessary to confirm the hemodynamic importance of aortic branch stenoses. Thin-cut computed tomographic arteriography (CTA) has improved the anatomic characterization of many complex lesions, and is currently the single most frequently used preoperative study.

Suprarenal abdominal aortic coarctations (n37), beginning above the celiac artery (CA) or superior mesenteric artery (SMA) included five patients with diffuse aortic hypoplasia, extending from the midthoracic aorta to the midabdominal aorta in three cases, and twice from the upper-most abdominal aorta to below the inferior mesenteric artery. In the later cases the narrowing was most severe in the upper abdominal aorta. Among suprarenal coarctations, all but four exhibited renal or splanchnic arterial stenoses or occlusions. *Intrarenal* coarctations (n12), beginning above the renal arteries, but below the SMA, were all associated with renal artery stenoses. *Infrarenal* coarctations (n4), beginning below the renal arteries, were focal in one case, presented as long tubular narrowings twice, and were associated with a terminal aortic occlusion once. Two of the four infrarenal coarctations exhibited renal artery stenoses.

Aortic Branch Disease. Renal artery stenoses affected 46 patients, being most often ostial (n44) and bilateral (n41). Aneurysms affected the proximal renal artery in three patients and the distal renal artery in one patient. Multiple renal arteries accompanied 43% of the suprarenal abdominal aortic coarctations. Splanchnic arterial disease included CA and SMA ostial stenoses or occlusions (n33), involving both vessels in all but six patients, as well as a CA aneurysm (n1) and common celiacomesenteric trunks (n4) of which one was aneurysmal.

Clinical Manifestations. Refractory hypertension was the major clinical manifestation, affecting 50 patients, whose mean preoperative blood pressure was 164/112 mmHg while on antihypertensive medications. Appropriate published age and gender-related standards for normal blood pressure were used in defining a child's blood pressure status. Hypertension was classified as *cured* if the patient was taking no antihypertensive medications and they were normotensive for the preceding six months; *improved* if they were normotensive while on drug therapy exclusive of angiotensin-converting enzyme (ACE) inhibitors, or if their diastolic pressure was higher than normal but 15% lower than preoperative levels; and *failures* if the diastolic pressure was higher than the normal and not 15% lower than preoperative levels or if ACE inhibitors were required for blood pressure control.

Three patients experienced intestinal angina with weight loss. Three additional patients described ischemia-related lower extremity fatigue with ambulation and had abnormal ankle-brachial indices that declined following treadmill exercise.

Surgical Treatment. Aortic reconstructions included thoracoabdominal bypasses, patch aortoplasties, and interposition aortoaortic grafts. No major therapeutic changes occurred over the decades of this study, with specific interventions, being dependent on the patient's age, and the pattern of the aortic disease as well as the associated renal and splanchnic arterial disease.

Thoracoabdominal bypass grafts (n26) were the most common intervention. These grafts originated from the distal thoracic aorta above the diaphragm or from the supraceliac aorta at the diaphragmatic hiatus,

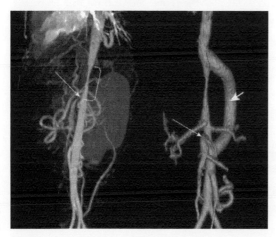

Thoracoabdominal bypass for a midabdomal aortic coarctation

being passed behind the left kidney to the terminal aorta. In most older patients, aortic exposure was facilitated by a thoracoabdominal incision through the left sixth or seventh intercostal space extending from the posterior axillary line across the costal margin, onto the abdomen, in either an oblique fashion to the right of the umbilicus or as a midline incision to just above the pubis. In younger children and adolescents, a transverse supraumbilical abdominal incision was used most often, extending laterally to the posterior axillary lines, combined with medial rotation of the viscera, allowing access to the abdominal aorta from its supraceliac level at the aortic hiatus to the origin of the iliac arteries.

Dacron knitted or woven thoracoabdominal grafts (n9) were used in the earlier experience, with expanded Teflon grafts (n17) used more often in recent years because of their greater stability regarding postimplantation dilatation. Graft diameter was chosen to be as big as possible, short of being so large that excessive luminal thrombus would accumulate. In children, the intent was always to oversize grafts compared to the aorta, with anticipated growth otherwise resulting in a graft too small to maintain normal distal pressures and flow. This translates into using 8–12 mm grafts in young children, 12–16 mm grafts for early adolescents, and 14–20 mm grafts in late adolescents and adults. In the very young child use of large conduits may not be possible. In the ideal circumstance, one should use a graft whose size would not represent an energy-consuming constriction as the patient grows into maturity. This means having a conduit at least 60% or 70% the size of the adult aorta. That is not always possible. Graft length was a non-issue in older children and adolescents, with axial growth from the diaphragm to pelvis being minimal after age 10.

Patch aortoplasty (n24) was usually undertaken when the coarctation segment had a large enough diameter to allow completion of the patch implantation without an overlap of sutures from the opposing sides of the patch. Whenever possible, patches in children were made sufficiently large enough, similar to thoracoabdominal graft sizing, so as to not be constrictive with growth into adulthood, yet not so generous as to risk development of an extensive lining of unstable thrombus. Teflon graft material was again favored over Dacron, because of the latter's propensity for dilatation years after implantation.

Interposition aortoaortic grafts (n3) were used in treating one

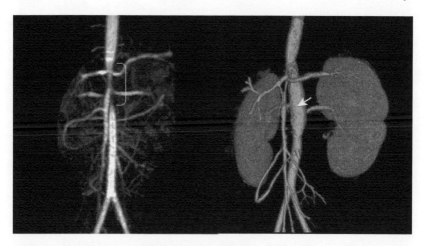

Patch aortoplasty for a midabdominal aortic coarctation

suprarenal and two infrarenal coarctations. The latter were placed using surgical techniques similar to those used in aortic aneurysm surgery. Exposure was through the retroperitoneum at the root of the mesocolon and small bowel mesentery, from the level of the left renal vein to the aortic bifurcation.

Primary renal and splanchnic arterial reconstructions were performed as simultaneous (n45) or staged (n13) procedures in relation to the patient's aortic surgery. When simultaneous reconstructions were performed, they usually were done following completion of the aortoplasty or aortic bypass. Among the staged operations, nine were prior to the aortic reconstruction, and four occurred after the aortic procedure. These nonaortic reconstructions included direct aortic implantations of the normal renal or splanchnic artery beyond the resected stenotic segment, as well as internal iliac aorto-visceral bypasses. Implantation of these arteries into a synthetic conduit or patch is not recommended because of the greater potential for later anastomotic narrowing. Four patients underwent a nephrectomy for unreconstructable renal artery disease, twice before the aortic procedure and two times at the time of the aortic reconstruction.

Operative Outcomes. No perioperative mortality followed the primary aortic or combined aortic and visceral arterial reconstructive procedures. Similarly, there were no ischemic intestinal complications or patients having postoperative renal insufficiency requiring dialysis. One patient with Moyamoya syndrome incurred a perioperative stroke but made a rapid recovery.

Early reoperations were performed without sequela for nonaortic-related complications, including intra-abdominal bleeding (n2), and a renal artery anastomotic pseudoaneurysm (n1). Life-table analysis documented excellent aortic graft patencies. Late reoperative aortic surgery occurred in two patients having thoracoabdominal bypasses. One outgrew the original graft and had a replacement graft seven years postoperatively, and the other underwent revision of a proximal anastomotic stenosis nine years postoperatively. Three patients with patch aortoplasties had late reoperations. Two with patches that proved inadequate in size with growth underwent thoracoabdominal bypasses, performed five and 10 years after their initial aortic procedure. The third patch failure, aneurysmal deterioration of the aorta at the site of the aortoplasty, occurred 14 years postoperatively and was treated with placement of an interposition aortoaortic graft.

Reoperations were anticipated in the three children who outgrew their original aortic reconstructions performed at ages five, six, and eight years. Their initial aortic procedure was considered essential for the child's health, could not be deferred to an older age, and could not safely have encompassed an initial aortic repair of greater dimensions. No perioperative mortality or major complications accompanied any of the aortic reoperations.

Thirty-nine of this series' patients had patent and satisfactory function of their visceral artery reconstructions (63 renal and 16 splanchnic individual revascularizations) at the latest time these vessels were imaged, averaging 5.4 years postoperative. Nine patients, including four of the former individuals and five additional patients, experienced failed visceral artery reconstructions (10 renal and 3 splanchnic revascularizations). These reconstructive failures included aneurysmal deterioration of four aortorenal vein bypass grafts, which are not used in contemporary practice. Eight patients with failed visceral reconstructions underwent successful reoperations five days to 12 years postoperatively, without mortality. The remaining patients' failed visceral reconstruction did not require reoperations.

Benefits of surgical therapy were reflected in cured (n28) or improved (n18) hypertension in 46 of the 53 patients. Their mean postoperative pressure was 121/72 mmHg at the most recent time of follow-up. This represented a significant decrease compared to the mean preoperative pressure (p<0.01). Four patients had no change in their hypertensive state and all were subjected to repeated operations, including two with secondary intraluminal stent placement (one aortic and one renal artery). The three patients with symptomatic lower extremity ischemia experienced complete relief following surgery. The three patients with intestinal angina had resolution of their postprandial abdominal pain and all had rapid weight gain.

Long-term follow-up of patients undergoing surgical treatment of their abdominal aortic coarctation is warranted. No patient in the present experience has developed an unacceptable failure of their aortic reconstruction. However, follow-up in this series has been relatively brief and has involved a generally younger group of patients with long life expectancies. Annual noninvasive assessments of lower extremity blood flow with exercise ankle-brachial indices are recommended. Imaging with MRA studies or CTA should be obtained if any evidence of diminished blood flow exists. Similar imaging is appropriate if blood pressure increases occur in those who have undergone concomitant renal artery reconstructions or whose renal blood flow is dependent upon their aortic reconstruction.

Six patients died late in follow-up, with none directly related to the patient's aortic disease or surgery. These deaths in patients ranging in age from 23 to 70 years occurred nine to 26 years postoperatively, and were due to trauma (n2), cancer (n2), stroke (n1), and myocardial infarction (n1). Contemporary follow-up was complete in all but four of the 47 surviving patients. Follow-up averaged 5.9 years. The patient's clinical status in the case of those individuals residing at long distances from the authors' hospital was obtained by direct contact with the referring physician.

We remain cautious at accepting the long-term benefits of endoluminal treatment of abdominal aortic coarctation in any patient, except in the older patient with very focal narrowings distant from their renal arteries. Given the high frequency with which the renal and splanchnic arteries are affected in abdominal aortic coarctation, especially in the younger-growing patient, lesions amenable to endovascular repair are likely to be limited.

In conclusion, abdominal aortic coarctation is uncommon and, and as evident in the present series, is often associated with coexisting splanchnic and renal artery occlusive disease. Carefully planned and executed surgical reconstructions of the aorta and involved branches will provide salutatory outcomes in more than 90% of these patients.

13

VISCERAL ARTERY ANEURYSMS

This work in a variety of forms and updates has been read multiple times at a University of California, Los Angeles Symposium on Vascular Diseases, including being included as the 2ⁿᵈ Wiley F. Barker Lecture on October 6, 1998, in Santa Monica, California. It has most recently been published as a chapter in Vascular and Endovascular Surgery: A Comprehensive Review, 8ᵗʰ edition, 695–707, W. S. Moore, editor, Philadelphia, Pennsylvania, Elsevier, 2013. The University of Michigan leadership in this field was established with two benchmark publications, one regarding splenic artery aneurysms (Surgery 74:898–909,1974) and the other regarding renal artery aneurysms (Ann Surg 234:454–463, 2001).

Splanchnic and renal artery aneurysms are uncommon, but with the introduction of newer imaging modalities they have become increasingly recognized in contemporary practice. Splanchnic artery aneurysms outnumber renal artery aneurysms 3:1. These two categories of visceral aneurysms deserve separate discussion. The University of Michigan has been a destination for many of these patients requiring treatment of their aneurysmal disease.

Twenty-two percent of splanchnic artery aneurysms present as emergencies, including 8.5% that result in death of the patient. More than half of those aneurysms reported in the English language literature have been described in the past 25 years. The anatomic distribution of these aneurysms has remained relatively constant in recent decades with the most common occurrence being in the splenic artery and the least common in the inferior mesenteric artery.

Splanchnic artery aneurysms represent a diversity of disease whose biologic character is often different and thus the method of treatment

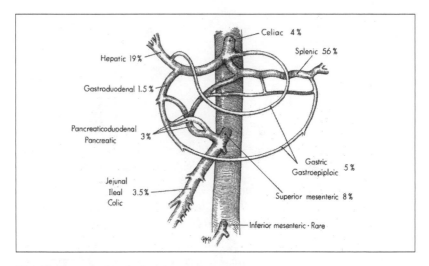

Distribution of splanchnic artery aneurysms

is different. In regard to treatment, many changes have occurred in the past five years. In most instances endovascular therapy is the preferred manner of treating these aneurysms, although open surgical therapy in select cases may be more appropriate. These aneurysms should be discussed individually.

Splenic Artery Aneurysms

Splenic artery aneurysms account for 60% of all splanchnic aneurysms, a percentage disproportion to the relative length of the artery at risk. Historically, female patients have outnumbered male patients 4:1, although in more recent years the female predilection appears to be less.

Many of these aneurysms are first noted on simple films of the abdomen with the presence of a signet-ring calcification. Calcific atherosclerosis is present in 70% of these aneurysms. CT, MRI, and conventional arteriography are the basis for most of these lesions being recognized in contemporary times.

The etiology of these lesions relates to a number of well-known and some less understood causes. Medial degeneration affects many of the women having these lesions, with 40% in the past literature having been grand multiparous with a history of six or more completed pregnancies. The marked increase in splenic artery blood flow during pregnancy and the hormonal effects on elastic tissues in the last trimester are considered contributors to these gestational-related aneurysms. There is often marked tortuosity of the splenic artery, which is characteristic of the affected vessel, especially in women who have had multiple pregnancies.

With the introduction of birth control in contemporary times, the 40% incidence of grand multiparity with these aneurysms has dropped to 10% in Western societies. Arterial fibrodysplasia affecting the renal arteries is accompanied by a 2% incidence of splenic aneurysms. Whether this is related to the patients being hypertensive or is a reflection of a generalized arteriopathy is unknown. Portal hypertension has been associated with a nearly 10% incidence of these aneurysms. In the case of portal hypertension, hyperdynamic flow exists within the portal-splanchnic system and increases in the splenic artery diameter correlate with increased size of these aneurysms. The hormonal changes associated with end-stage cirrhosis associated with portal hypertension likely contribute to the formation of these lesions.

Inflammation as a cause of these aneurysms is usually pancreatitis-related with pseudocyst erosion into the splenic artery. Both blunt and penetrating abdominal trauma are less common causes of these aneurysms. Arteriosclerosis is present in many aneurysms but is considered a secondary, not a primary causative event. The fact is that such atherosclerotic changes in the wall of these aneurysms represent a ubiquitous phenomenon affecting many other aneurysms throughout the body. Calcified atherosclerotic changes often occur within the aneurysm but not within the adjacent vessel. Multiple bland aneurysms are noted in 20% of patients. Those with portal hypertension have an even greater frequency of multiplicity.

Splenic artery aneurysm rupture has been reported to affect 2% of bland lesions with a 25% mortality. An exception exists with pregnancy; 95% of aneurysms diagnosed during pregnancy have ruptured with a 70% maternal mortality and 75% fetal mortality. Although the rupture rates appear exceedingly high with pregnancy it is likely that many patients have asymptomatic lesions during earlier gestations that

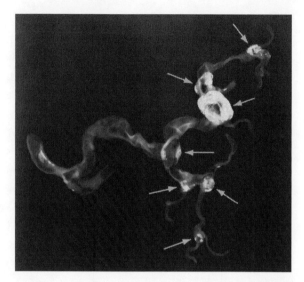

Splenic artery aneurysms occurring at each branch point of the artery

simply go recognized. It is of note that the rupture rate and mortality is doubled with bland aneurysms occurring in patients with portal hypertension.

Bland aneurysms that rupture may bleed first into the lesser sac and then continue bleeding into the peritoneal cavity causing the so-called "double rupture" phenomena. Pancreatitis-related splenic aneurysms are often associated with pseudocyst erosion into the arteries and stomach, causing gastrointestinal hemorrhage rather than free intraperitoneal bleeding.

The operative indications include interventions in all childbearing females; all symptomatic cases (it is of note that 20% of patients having these aneurysms experience abdominal discomfort, albeit difficult to relate such to the aneurysm per se); and bland aneurysms greater than 2 cm in diameter if the surgical mortality is less than 0.5% (the latter representing the product of the 2% predicted rupture rate of bland aneurysms and known 25% mortality following such).

Operative intervention for noninflammatory aneurysms is most often endovascular embolization. Bland splenic artery aneurysms are quite favorably treated by endovascular occlusion. Coil embolization, in particular for more distal aneurysms near the splenic parenchyma, is appropriate. More proximal lesions may be treated with simple plugs or stent grafts in select patients to isolate the aneurysm. The presence of a ruptured aneurysm resulting in an arteriovenous fistula is also ideal for an endovascular intervention.

Open splenectomy or obliteration and excision of the aneurysm is usually performed for failures of catheter-based interventions. Multiple intraparenchymal aneurysms will require a plethora of coils with predictable postembolization splenic infarction and symptoms referable to such. The frequent tortuosity of the splenic artery may make catheterization of some distal lesions more difficult. In both the former settings, one may have to resort to an open procedure.

Similarly, aneurysms due to pseudocyst erosion, which affect nearly 10% of individuals with chronic alcoholic pancreatitis, may require an open operation. Treatment of these aneurysms by distal pancreatectomy with removal of the spleen is clearly definitive therapy.

Hepatic Artery Aneurysms

Hepatic artery aneurysms account for 20% of splanchnic aneurysms with a male predilection of 2:1 being somewhat less evident in more contemporary practice. Half of these patients have other splanchnic aneurysms.

The most common cause is related to abdominal trauma (such as high-speed motor vehicle accidents with pseudoaneurysms recognized on CT scans obtained during the evaluation of this trauma), as well as percutaneous hepatobiliary procedures. Medial degeneration is a second cause that has been present in approximately 20% of these aneurysms. Mycotic lesions, which were quite common in the early part of the last century, account for less than 10% of contemporary encounters. Arteriosclerosis, as has been the case with splenic aneurysms, is considered a secondary event. These aneurysms are extrahepatic in 80% of cases, with 20% being intrahepatic. The former are usually solitary.

Hepatic artery aneurysm rupture has been reported historically to occur in 20% of these cases, and carries a mortality of 35%. Contemporary rates of both these events are somewhat less. Most of these lesions are asymptomatic, and when they do become symptomatic the majority are greater than 3 cm in diameter. With rupture, hemorrhage occurs equally into the biliary tract (especially with traumatic lesions) and into the peritoneal cavity. The former is a recognized cause of hematobilia with its associated biliary colic, hematemesis, and jaundice.

Operative indications for hepatic artery aneurysms include intervening on asymptomatic extrahepatic aneurysms that exceed 2 cm in diameter and select intrahepatic lesions, as well as all symptomatic lesions.

Hepatic artery aneurysms are preferentially managed by endovascular occlusion with or without stent graft placement, depending on the particular vessel involved and the adequacy of the liver's collateral circulation. Resection or exclusion with or without arterial reconstruction may be undertaken in select cases as well as aneurysmorrhaphy in some cases of penetrating trauma. Hepatic territory resection is only undertaken for uncontrolled life-threatening hemorrhage and is very uncommon.

Superior Mesenteric Artery Aneurysms

Superior mesenteric artery aneurysms account for 5.5% of these splanchnic lesions with a male:female ratio of 2 to 1. Mycotic lesions continue to be common with infection, usually due to septic emboli from endocarditis with beta-hemolytic strept organisms being most frequently encountered. Medial degeneration has been associated most often with dissections. Like the aneurysms previously mentioned, atherosclerosis, which occurs in 20% of these lesions, is considered a secondary event.

Rupture of these aneurysms occurs with an undefined frequency, although a 10% figure is reasonable. Dissections often result in a large mural hematoma with compression of the true lumen of the vessel. Occlusion, frequently occurring with a dissection, may involve obstruction of the inferior pancreaticoduodenal and middle colic vessels and leave the small bowel at risk for profound ischemia. Such is the basis for the prodromata of intestinal angina in many of these individuals. The indications for operation include symptomatic aneurysms, bland aneurysms greater than 1.5 cm diameter, and select dissections.

Operative intervention is most often ligation and aneurysmectomy with or without a reconstruction of the vessel. In select cases endovascular stent graft placement is appropriate.

Celiac Artery Aneurysms

Celiac artery aneurysms account for 4% of all splanchnic aneurysms and are most often associated with medial degeneration. The proximal celiac trunk is usually not involved with the aneurysm. Arteriosclerosis again is a secondary event and mycotic aneurysms, which were noted in the early history of these lesions, are rarely seen today. There is no gender predilection. Most occur as a saccular aneurysm affecting the distal trunk of the celiac artery. Associated abdominal aortic aneurysms are present in 20% of cases, and 40% have other splanchnic aneurysms. Most of these aneurysms are asymptomatic.

Celiac artery aneurysm rupture has been reported in approximately 13% of contemporary cases with a mortality of 50%. Earlier reports suggested a near 80% mortality, usually associated with exsanguinating intraperitoneal bleeding heralded by a very brief period of epigastric and severe back pain

Operative intervention in good risk patients is recommended for

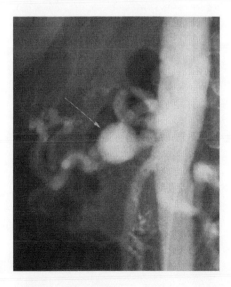

Celiac artery aneurysm

aneurysms exceeding 2 cm in diameter. Endovascular procedures are less invasive and may be undertaken if significant branch involvement does not exist and the patient has a good collateral circulation to the foregut. Otherwise an open aneurysmectomy with a possible arterial reconstruction is preferable. Surprisingly, ligation and resection without reconstruction is often undertaken without major complications. Simple preservation of the foregut circulation with a hepatosplenic reanastomosis following excision of the aneurysm would be the least of the open procedures to be undertaken.

Gastric And Gastroepiploic Artery Aneurysms

Gastric artery and gastroepiploic artery aneurysms account for 4% of these splanchnic lesions with a male to female ratio of 2 to 1. Gastric aneurysms are 10 times more common than gastroepiploic aneurysms. They are often quite small and difficult to recognize without careful imaging. Most of these aneurysms are acquired, being associated with medial degeneration or periarterial inflammation from associated bowel disease.

Rupture has affected 90% of reported cases, with gastrointestinal bleeding being twice as common as intraperitoneal bleeding. Most of those patients experiencing rupture have few antecedent symptoms, and rupture carries a mortality of 70%. This would suggest that once recognized these aneurysms should all be treated.

Operative intervention for extraintestinal lesions can be undertaken with ligation with or without aneurysmectomy. For those intramural lesions causing gastrointestinal bleeding, aneurysmectomy with gastric tissue excision is appropriate. Endovascular intervention for these lesions may be lifesaving in cases of severe hemorrhage, although an open procedure is likely to be required soon thereafter.

Jejunal, Ileal, And Colic Artery Aneurysms

Jejunal, ileal, and colic artery aneurysms account for 3% of these splanchnic lesions with no gender predilection. They are most often noted as incidental findings on imaging obtained for other nonvascular diseases.

Rupture is considered uncommon with bleeding occurring equally into the mesentery, intestinal lumen, and peritoneal cavity. It is of some note that a more recent report has suggested a 30% rupture rate with a 20% mortality, albeit this likely represents a unique experience. Treatment usually involves simple ligation of the affected artery and occasionally an aneurysmectomy with possible bowel resection. Endovascular interventions with embolic occlusion of these lesions are appropriate when bleeding is exsanguinating, but most of these individuals will require an exploration following such control.

Gastroduodenal and Pancreaticoduodenal Artery Aneurysms

Gastroduodenal artery aneurysms as well as pancreaticoduodenal and pancreatic artery aneurysms account for 1.5 and 2% of splanchnic aneurysms, respectively. In general these are the most difficult to treat of all splanchnic aneurysms because of their location. Males outnumber females, 4 to 1. Two causes are responsible for most of these aneurysms. Medial degeneration is common with high flow in those arteries acting as collaterals in patients with a celiac artery occlusion. Among flow-related aneurysms the gastroduodenal artery is affected in 10% of cases and the pancreaticoduodenal artery in 90%. Inflammation pancreatitis-related aneurysms are the second type that account for 50% of gastroduodenal aneurysms and 30% of pancreaticoduodenal aneurysms.

Most of these aneurysms have been recognized on simple imaging studies. Many have been associated with celiac artery narrowings. Selective SMA injections in these cases will demonstrate celiac artery stenosis or occlusion with a bird's-beak V formed by the common hepatic and splenic vessels with no evidence of any flow within the proximal celiac artery. It is believed that these aneurysms evolve due to the excessively high flow through the pancreaticoduodenal and gastroduodenal collateral circulations between the superior mesenteric and celiac circulations.

In other instances these aneurysms are pancreatitis-related. Some aneurysms affecting the inferior pancreaticoduodenal artery in the head of the pancreas may be associated with obstructive biliary tract

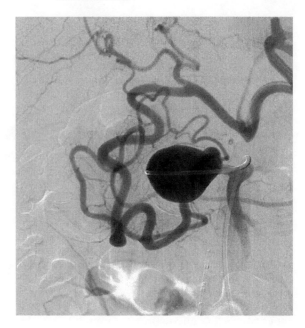

Inferior pancreati-
coduodenal artery
aneurysm

symptoms. They obviously represent a significant diagnostic as well as therapeutic challenge. These pancreatitis-related lesions are much more difficult to treat than those associated with a simple medial degenerative process.

Rupture has been reported in 30 to 50% of these aneurysms. Bleeding occurs 85% of the time into the gastrointestinal tract and 15% into the peritoneal cavity. The reported mortality following rupture is 50%; albeit this often is a reflection of spectacular cases described in the literature. The actual mortality accompanying rupture is more likely to be 20% affecting the gastroduodenal artery and 10% when the pancreaticoduodenal artery is involved in patients having celiac artery occlusions.

Operative intervention is recommended in the vast majority of these patients, with endovascular occlusion often being the initial therapy, especially in patients with life-threatening hemorrhage, to be followed by a later open procedure in the case of patients with pancreatitis-related disease, including a simple ligation within the pseudoaneurysm sac, or pancreatic resection, including a pancreaticoduodenectomy in rare cases. Open intervention with an aneurysmectomy and possible vessel reconstruction may be more appropriate in those patients with celiac occlusion having aneurysms affecting their collateral circulation. Open surgery allows recognition of ischemic changes within the liver and foregut structures, which if severe warrant a reconstruction to restore celiac blood flow.

Inferior Mesenteric Artery Aneurysms

Inferior mesenteric artery aneurysms are rare, with 49 of these having been reported in the English literature including 18 in the past two years. These have multiple etiologies, including aneurysmal development when the artery serves as a major collateral in patients with SMA and CA occlusive disease. In general their natural history is unknown, but when diagnosed operative intervention is recommended, usually with simple ligation of the vessel, except in those cases when the inferior mesenteric vessel acts as important conduit for blood to the mid and foregut circulations. Then a reconstruction is necessary.

True Renal Artery Macroaneurysms

Renal artery macroaneurysms are uncommon with a reported incidence of approximately 0.1% as evident in more than 8,500 arteriograms for nonvascular disease obtained at the University of Michigan. The frequency of these lesions increases to 0.7% in patients having hypertension and 9.2% in those that have fibrodysplasia affecting the renal vessels. The latter likely accounts for the slight predominance of female to male patients with a ratio of 1.2 to 1.

The majority are saccular with 90% being extrarenal and 10% intrarenal. Primary or secondary branchings are affected in 75% of cases. Most of these aneurysms are asymptomatic as was the case in 252 aneurysms affecting 168 patients reported from the University of Michigan. These lesions are most often recognized as incidental findings, with calcification on a plain abdominal film or with other imaging modalities such as CT or MRA. Conventional arteriography is most useful at defining the specific anatomy in most cases, although thin-cut CTA is of near equal value.

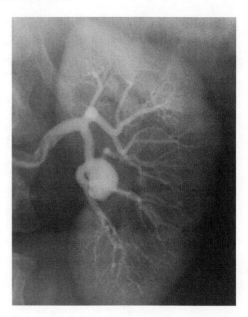

Renal artery aneurysm

The majority of these aneurysms appear to result from a congenital discontinuity of the internal elastic lamina with an associated medial degenerative process. Many of these aneurysms are comprised of nothing but a fibrous wall with few cellular abnormalities, with evidence elsewhere in the aneurysm of focal cholesterol clefts and calcification representing the expected secondary arteriosclerotic phenomena.

Clinical manifestations of true renal aneurysms are few and the vast majority of these patients are asymptomatic. Although 80% of individuals with these aneurysms have elevated blood pressure, only a small percentage of them are thought to have hypertension because of the aneurysm, per se. Rupture has occurred in 3% of reported cases. Among the few having hypertension thought due to their aneurysm, embolization may have occurred into the smaller segmental vessels resulting in a segment of ischemic kidney. A rare patient may torque the renal artery exiting the aneurysm and cause the pressure within the kidney to fall and contribute to renin release and hypertension.

Covert rupture is one of the two forms of rupture affecting renal aneurysms. Covert rupture into an adjacent vein results in a large arteriovenous fistula, which may be associated with hematuria and hypertension. Death is a very rare accompaniment. Covert rupture has been reported in a little less than 2% of those cases described in the literature.

Overt rupture has also been reported in nearly 2% of cases in the literature, with loss of the kidney occurring in 90% of individuals and death in 10%. Pregnancy represents an exception, with rupture carrying a risk of maternal death in 50% and fetal death in 75% of cases. Overt rupture is usually an operative or postmortem diagnosis, or occasionally following arteriographic studies where there is nonvisualization of the kidney and accumulation of peripelvic contrast. Clearly with no parenchymal blood flow after one hour of normothermic ischemia, irreparable renal injury may occur, and salvage of the kidney will be limited.

Operative indications for the treatment of renal artery aneurysms include any patient who is symptomatic, those who have coexistent renovascular hypertension, all childbearing aged females, and when the size is greater than 3 cm (assuming the interventionist is experienced).

Operative intervention includes renal revascularization, endovascular occlusion of the aneurysm with its attendant risk of renal infarction, and lastly nephrectomy in the case of irreparable renal ischemia.

In the case of open surgery, we prefer a transverse abdominal incision with a reflection of the viscera to allow exposure of the great vessels as well as the distal renal vasculature. Such an exposure allows one to perform nearly a bench-like reconstruction of the renal artery. We favor resection of large secular aneurysms with a primary angioplastic closure of the arterial defect and an occasional use of vein graft patch if needed. In those individuals who have coexisting fibrodysplasia, the vessel should be reconstructed after the aneurysmectomy using an autologous bypass graft.

In conclusion, aneurysms affecting the splanchnic and renal arteries have differing etiologies and clinical manifestations. Their treatment requires differing interventions dependent upon the artery involved and the cause of the aneurysm.

PATIENT-CENTRIC CARE

Large multispecialty clinics and major medical centers have an obligation to provide thorough and efficient care. The past practice of individual assessments, one after another, undertaken by a plethora of physicians—. frequently specialists often having little time to communicate with each other—is a perverse form of medicine. At best it delays timely treatment and in nearly all circumstances it drives up health-care costs.

Patients should be removed from the periphery of multiple specialists and become the central focus of the specialists' care where they will hear one voice as to their diagnostic or treatment options. The University of Michigan Cardiovascular Center was created to support patient-centric care rather than a specialty-centric arc of care. The result has trumped all prior practice patterns.

14

THE CARDIOVASCULAR CENTER:
GROUNDBREAKING

These remarks were read at the Groundbreaking Ceremony of the University of Michigan's Cardiovascular Center on September 5, 2003, in Ann Arbor, Michigan.

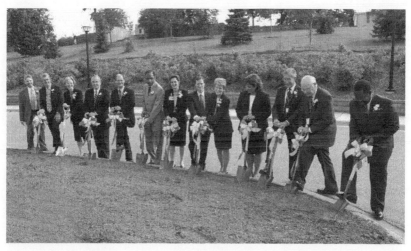

Groundbreaking for the University of Michigan Cardiovascular Center, 2003. Those present (left to right) included: David Pinsky-Chief Cardiovascular Medicine, Alan Lichter-Medical School Dean, Elizabeth Nabel-Director NIH Heart, Lung and Blood Institute, The Author-Head Vascular Surgery, Kim Eagle-Head Clinical Cardiology, Larry Warren-Chief Executive Officer University Hospital, Linda Larin-Chief Administrative Officer CVC, Timothy Slottow-University Executive Vice President and Chief Financial Officer, Mary Sue Coleman-University President, Stephanie Diccion-McDonald-Director Nursing CVC, Lazar Greenfield-Interim University Vice President Medical Affairs, Robert Kelch-Vice President Emeritus Medical Affairs, Anthony Denton-Chief Operating Officer University Hospital.

We are gathered here today because those in our past have had the vision and faith that a Center such as this is the right thing for patients, for the University of Michigan, for our time, and for the future. The Cardiovascular Center began nearly a decade ago as a grassroots up idea by many faculty, both clinicians and scientists. It received the blessing of the University Officers and Regents as a virtual Center in 2000, and in the spring of 2003 they approved Phase I of the Center—the clinical facility, for which we celebrate the groundbreaking today. Phase II, our research laboratories, is in the planning stage.

Although the Center is a contemporary idea, as a concept it has its roots in the history of cardiovascular care at the University—and that history is indeed a rich one. Many individuals have gained worldwide recognition for contributing to our understanding of cardiovascular diseases. Let me mention a few.

Perhaps the dominant contribution during the last century was that of Frank Wilson, an erudite and mathematically oriented leader of our cardiologists, who nearly 75 years ago developed the unipolar lead and revolutionized the EKG, allowing for the accurate diagnosis of heart attacks and other diseases of the heart. Nine of the 12 leads in EKGs used everywhere were of Dr. Wilson's doing.

Then, with the ability to surgically bypass obstructed coronary arteries, there came the need to bypass the heart and lung to allow for open heart surgery. Although Gibbons in Philadelphia was the first to devise the bypass machine, it was in Ann Arbor that Richard Sarns, an engineer, more than four decades ago perfected the heart-lung machine. In fact, the Sarns' machine was used by Christian Bernard in 1967, during the 1st heart transplant in Cape Town, South Africa, and is used today in more than 80% of open heart procedures. Many of our cardiac surgeons worked on this effort, including some of us as undergraduate students at the University of Michigan.

Nowhere but in children with congenital heart disease has open heart surgery been more successful—and no one helped better establish pediatric cardiac surgery than had Herbert Sloan, who headed our Cardiac Surgery Service for nearly two decades and was the first to report 100 survivors following surgery for tetralogy of Fallot, by all accounts, to this day one of the classic papers in cardiac surgery.

Then came the catheter-based therapies for patients with heart attacks. Eric Topol and his cadre of Michigan cardiologists, was at the forefront in treating these patients with lytic therapy and balloon angioplasty. Most senior faculty can remember his lead article in the *New England Journal of Medicine* describing the successful treatment of many elderly patients in cardiogenic shock who previously were treated by bed rest, and of whom many died. How many of you can recall seeing the helicopter ferry a critically ill patient from a neighboring ER to our cath labs with a brown paper bag labeled "tPA" study? Those were exciting times!

During this same time period, the risk factors contributing to heart and vascular disease were being better understood. The role of smoking was better defined by Maurice Seevers, the Chairman of Pharmacology, who was a major contributor to the first Surgeon General's report on the hazards of cigarettes, and the importance of managing high blood pressure was better defined by Sibley Hoobler and Stevo Ju_lius. Dr. Hoobler had established the second Division of Hypertension in the country. One outcome of the efforts of Drs. Hoobler and Julius was to recognize renal artery obstruction as the most common cause of correctable hypertension, a disease whose anatomic and hemodynamic features were best defined by Joseph Bookstein, a radiologist and the founder of our Angiography division. The first aortorenal bypass performed to treat this disease was undertaken in "Old Main," our former University Hospital, by Bill DeWeese, who as a medical student was my attending staff, mentor, and hero.

In addition to these clinical contributions, many fundamental and early concepts of cardiac and vascular function and disease were forthcoming from the basic scientists of our medical school, including Ben Lucchesi and David Bohr. Ben was a classmate of mine who was also a Pharmacology Professor; his early work on arrhythmias included the first paper, written over 40 years ago, on the anti-arrhythmic use of beta-blockers. David Bohr was a physiologist whose experiments on vascular smooth muscle reactivity gave great insight into the causes of hypertension. These two were stellar scientists.

The accomplishments of the earlier days are easily defined; however, it is sometimes harder to put present-day accomplishments into perspective. Nevertheless, the work of Betsy Nabel on gene transfer and expression in the vessel wall represented the first time a living intact animal had a transplanted gene function. This work, published in *Science* in 1989, will stand the test of time.

We have a remarkable group of forebearers. All have a common theme: inquiry, discovery, and application to the human condition. That is our legacy and our challenge—research and clinical care.

To explore the human condition through research, with an awareness that your work may improve humankind and with the opportunity to teach our successors about this experience, is the essence of being a university professor; the sense of belonging has its roots in the history of our institution, and those who have contributed to our heritage in the past should be proud of this unique Center to be built on our campus. We are indeed among the very fortunate in our profession.

Thank you

15

THE CARDIOVASCULAR CENTER:
GRAND OPENING

The celebratory grand opening of the Cardiovascular Center occurred on June 7, 2007, on a very warm day in the garden area of the Center. Remarks were made by University President Mary Sue Coleman; the Vice President for Medical Affairs, Robert Kelch; the Center directors; a patient, Eric Morganroth; and two distinguished alumni of our medical school and postgraduate residency programs, Sanjay Gupta (CNNs chief medical correspondent and a practicing neurosurgeon) and Antonio Novello (US Surgeon General in the first Bush administration, and currently the New York State Health Commissioner). The author felt he had one of the prized opportunities at the podium—to welcome the hundreds before us, and to introduce Mary Sue Coleman and Sanjay Gupta.

One of my greatest pleasures has been to serve with Rich Prager, David Pinsky, and Kim Eagle as a CVC Director. The four of us along with Linda Larin, our chief administrative officer, welcome you to today's opening ceremony, particularly our patients, our families, many university executives, staff and faculty, including Regents, governmental officials, our builders and the wonderful architects of this facility, and especially the many benefactors who have made this such a special place.

And a special place it is; indeed, more than 400 of you contributed to the planning of the Center. And you know, you got it right. It is a wonderful visual respite—for hope and healing. The light, the art, and the ambiance are disarmingly peaceful, and it is a maze of some of the most spectacular medical technology you can imagine.

But what really makes this special are the CVC people and their four core values. First, we care about respect and compassion; we really

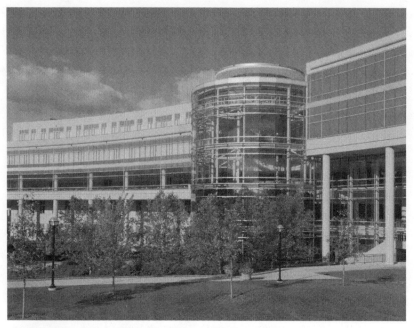

The University of Michigan Cardiovascular Center, 2007

honor and care for one another as individuals. Second, we care about collaboration; we honor the synergy of team, built on trust. Third, we care about innovation; we vigorously honor both individual and collective creativity. And fourth, we are committed to excellence; we truly honor the intrinsic desire to be leaders and to be the best.

Our master-of-ceremonies this afternoon is Dr. Sanjay Gupta. Sanjay earned his undergraduate and medical degrees from the University of Michigan, and completed his residency training here. He is a member of the CVC's National Advisory Board. Most of you never saw him as a student or trainee, but you certainly have seen him on TV. Dr. Gupta joined CNN in the summer of 2001 and he has become an icon in the medical news field, providing knowledge and hope to millions from disparate corners of our globe. His impact on health care has been felt by many here—and many in less advantaged lands. In that role he has been a priceless American ambassador, and for this we are in his debt. He's got it together.

Let me be somewhat personal and quote excerpts from one letter among many that we dredged from our files, written about him when he was seeking a surgical residency after attending our medical school.

"Sanjay is a very unique young man who has demonstrated great maturity and outstanding intellect as he has pursued his academic career. Sanjay is a very pleasant and highly motivated student who has a good sense of humor and is highly respected by his peers as well as teachers. His intenseness was masked by a gentle personality when relating to patients, their families, fellow students, and the residents with whom he was working. Perhaps the most unique characteristic of Sanjay Gupta is his clear success as a leader. He does not appear to be driven to achievement-oriented positions, but rather seems to be the type of individual that both superiors and subordinates turn to when group decisions are being made. He is a joy to work with."

Pretty nice comments about a senior medical student. When I was a younger faculty member I had the wonderful opportunity to mentor Sanjay as a student and junior surgical resident, and in fact the quotes I've just recited are from a letter I authored more than 15 years ago. You

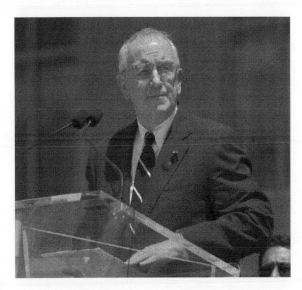

The author addressing those attending the CVC opening

know, being a university faculty member includes the fun of teaching bright young students, but the real reward is seeing them make a difference in our world after they graduate. Sanjay Gupta has done that.

Welcome home, Sanjay.

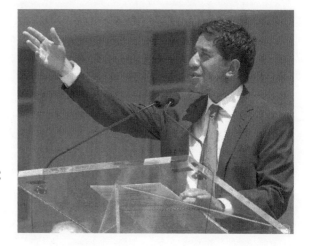

Sanjay Gupta
addressing the
audience at the CVC
opening ceremony

16

PATIENT-CENTRIC VERSUS
SPECIALTY-CENTRIC CARE:
THE MICHIGAN DIFFERENCE

This address was read before the 6th Annual Western Vascular Institute Symposium on May 29, 2008, in Galway, Ireland. A similar formal presentation by the author occurred in Dubrovnik, Croatia, on October 1, 2009, and on other occasions at many academic medical centers in the United States.

The University of Michigan is very proud to have established a broad-reaching practice and business model of cardiovascular care that favors patient-centric care and disfavors professional turf battles and the silo practices seen in the past. The Cardiovascular Center is a unique and special place with an exceptional group of Medical Directors who share equally in its management: Kim Eagle, David Pinsky, Richard Prager, and myself, all with the guidance of Linda Larin, who is our Chief Administrative Director.

The Center carries forth with a deep commitment to its core values. They have great value in pursuing our mission and receive support from a very different governance organization.

The Center does not have a single director. It has four directors representing the principal specialties of the Center, and each has an equal voice in determining operational policy, investing in programs, and developing a strategic plan. They all hold academic appointments in traditional Departments, but their appointments as a Center Director come jointly from the Medical School Dean and University Hospital Executive Director.

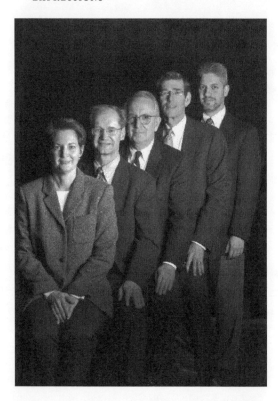

The CVC Leadership:
Linda Larin, Kim Eagle,
the author, Richard
Prager, David Pinsky

The Directors as physicians are committed to change the paradigm of how cardiovascular care is provided. Our obligation is to pursue seminal research into preventing and treating cardiovascular disease, and to offer compassionate care at the boundaries of contemporary medicine. Make no mistake about it—this means providing patient-centric care. Specialty-centric competition and conflict in the care of vascular disease has been recognized for decades to be a common cause of dysfunctional professional efforts and a source of increasing health-care costs in the United States.

For many years the University of Michigan Hospital had been a major referral center with a long-standing reputation of expertise in the traditional care of patients with cardiovascular disease. However, as service line care became important in providing efficient and effective care for specific diseases, a commitment to a multispecialty center evolved. In 2000 a virtual Cardiovascular Center within the University Hospital was approved by the University's Board of Regents. They also approved moving forward with the planning of a new facility to be the hub of a new Cardiovascular Center.

Over the next two years, the Center directors, representing cardiology, cardiac surgery, and vascular surgery, with the Center's administrative director, worked with many who were responsible for producing the architectural plans for the Center's building. The Regents then approved construction of the new Center and ground was broken in 2003.

In 2007 the 350,000-square-foot freestanding Cardiovascular Center opened. It encompassed physicians' offices, conference rooms, 36 clinic rooms, 14 invasive laboratories, 10 surgical suites, 24 ICU beds, and 24 inpatient beds for the vascular surgery patients. Cardiology and cardiac surgery inpatient beds remained in the adjacent University Hospital connected by an elevated walkway at the fourth level above ground. The facility was quite open with a large six-story atrium with patient wait-areas looking onto a garden below. All patient rooms were private, both in the intensive care unit on one level, and the vascular surgery unit beds on a second level. The operating rooms were state-of-the-art; three with fully operational imaging equipment.

The Cardiovascular Center houses more than 230 full-time physicians and scientists from the disciplines of vascular surgery, cardiac surgery, cardiology, interventional radiology, stroke neurology, and cardiovascular anesthesiology.

The annual Cardiovascular Center activity encompasses over 50,000 outpatient visits, 7,000 admissions, 142,000 noninvasive procedures, 1,400 open heart procedures, and close to 4,000 vascular surgery and endovascular interventions. In 2008 this activity generated $225 million dollars in net revenue, including a $67 million margin.

The Cardiovascular Center faculty and staff have had a unique opportunity to advance our understanding of and treatment of cardiovascular diseases through the funding of diverse innovative clinical, educational, and research projects. Monies for these projects are distributed by the Directors from a $50 million philanthropic fund. This large gift was received from an anonymous benefactor who requested that we "eliminate the old practice patterns of specialty-oriented care." These monies are distributed solely by the four Center Directors, independent of hospital or medical school administration, including Departmental Chairs.

The Center Directors also established ten collaborative teams, including (1) Vascular and Endovascular Surgery, (2) Cardiovascular Imaging, (3) Cardiac Surgery-Invasive Cardiology, (4) Arrhythmia, (5) Heart Failure-Transplant, (6) Inpatient Care, (7) Outpatient Care, (8) Clinical Research, (9) Basic Research, and (10) Education. All teams have been financially incented to develop innovative projects of their own choice that elevates their stature as clinicians and scientists.

Scholarly programs funded by the Directors have resulted in robust research productivity in the past 2 ½ years with 1,243 publications; 32 new patents; and a total of direct research funding of $116.5 million, including indirect funding of an additional $42 million. Funding from the National Institutes of Health totaled $92 million, with nonfederal funding accounting for the remainder.

The physicians of the Cardiovascular Center have accepted the basic tenet that financial issues separating specialty practices are often a source of contention—and not always in the patient's best interest. Incenting individuals across disciplines to combine their expertise has enhanced seamless patient-centric care and made the University of Michigan Cardiovascular Center's organizational model successful. Perhaps an important link in the success is the fact that the Directors, representing the principal specialties, serve as equal partners in developing and executing all strategic plans. Their collegial collaboration is a template for all members of the Cardiovascular Center, regardless of their diverse specialties. Many institutions from throughout the United States have made site visits to gain an understanding of what the Michigan Difference is all about. We are a proud Cardiovascular Center.

Addendum: Palpable enthusiasm surrounded the faculty and staff who entered the new Cardiovascular Center in 2007. In part, this represented the well-known uplifting spirit when moving into a spacious new place with friends. But it was more than that. It was a realization that what they were doing in their professional lives had enough value that the University had invested many millions of dollars in creating a truly exceptional building for them to practice and work in.

Equally important was receipt of one of the University's largest philanthropic gifts from an anonymous donor. That gift of $50 million gave the Center's members a visible degree of independence from the competing interests of the rest of the Health System. It was perhaps this gift, and its attendant independence, that more than anything else differentiates the Cardiovascular Center from other patient-centric groups in our own Hospital as well as throughout the Nation.

For nearly six years, the Center Directors and University Executive Officers kept their promise to keep the donors name anonymous. It was a silence difficult to keep quiet about—the gift directed to a new paradigm of cardiovascular care had no equal amongst our peers—but silence was kept with great respect. Then on March 21, 2014, the Center was formally named "The Samuel and Jean Frankel Cardiovascular Center," and the children of this generous couple, through a family foundation, were recognized as the donors. This transformative gift, to be distributed over two decades, continues to strengthen the unique multispecialty leadership structure of the Center and gives daily emphasis to our core values and commitment to patient-centered care.

PROFESSORSHIPS

There is something of value in thought and deed to a college or university when it invites an individual into the professorial ranks. It's more than a simple job to those entering at the most junior level, carrying the potential to advance to higher levels with accompanying tenure. But a conventional appointment pales in comparison to receiving a "Named Professorship," which carries prestige to the granting institution and a modicum of independence to the recipient to pursue scholarly projects unencumbered with the usual responsibilities of one's job.

At the University of Michigan, named professorships are endowed and once established will persist as long as the University exists. When, like the author, you are honored to receive one of these professorships and even more honored to have the University create one in your name, it must be considered the apogee of one's professional career.

17

BOUNDARIES:

THE HANDLEMAN PROFESSORSHIP

This address was read at the University of Michigan inauguration of the Marion and David Handleman Professorship in Vascular Surgery on July 13, 2005, in Ann Arbor, Michigan. The author was the recipient of the Professorship.

This professorship means more to me than any other academic accolade you might imagine. To be honored with a named professorship is a remarkable benchmark that few receive and something to be held close to one's academic core values. Such has been so for me.

My thoughts these past few days have been centered on boundaries—including those that we must pass through to better understand ourselves and improve the human condition.

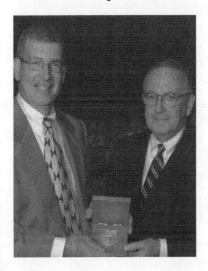

Dean Alan Lichter and the author, with the University's medallion medal recognizing the establishment of the Handleman Professorship

There are some boundaries that are seemingly not definable, like the limits of our universe, but standard definitions of a boundary do exist, two of which are quite dissimilar. One refers to something that indicates limits, like staying within bounds; you may be safe but your view will always be limited. The other defines a frontier, where new perspectives exist. This is where research resides and succeeds. I believe my parents, teachers, mentors, and especially the University have had a covenant to provide safety within boundaries, but they also have had an obligation to aid the young in leaving their comfort zone at the boundary so that they may discover new worlds that will inspire, in both thought and substance.

My core family took this serious, both my parents and my brother. My mother represented a Midwestern educated woman who grew up in Ohio but went to college in Boston and my brother, Bob, attended art school at Parsons in New York City. They both allowed me to express myself by being creative in both drawing and writing.

My father, a successful busi- nessman involved with munici- pal securities, was a real "guy": a great sportsman, a profes- sional basketball player in the 1920's—and the author of some of my earliest boundaries. First, no "gentleman's Cs." He simply refused to allow me to accept being average, but he never pushed me. Second, I, like all kids, wanted a new mitt or ball every year, and his admonition that "equipment doesn't make the athlete" stung, but you know he was right. Lastly, he often let me step beyond the boundary— buying a car when I was only 15, too young to even have a driv- er's license; leaving engineering

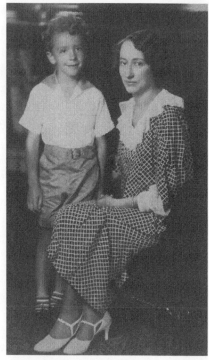

My mother, Jeannette, and brother, Bob, c. 1936

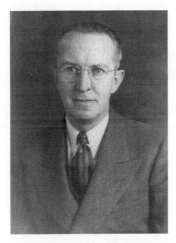

My father, Dean, c 1956

school to become a premed student my sophomore year; and as many times I've heard that the "equipment doesn't make the athlete" I heard "I trust your judgment."

At age eight I used to listen to 15-minute broadcasts from Antarctica by Richard E. Byrd. Those times encouraged me to think out of my own backyard. Then at age nine my father took me to Fairchild Theatre on the campus of Michigan State College to hear the Admiral, who had explored both poles. He revealed that beyond the boundaries are wonders and hardship and nothing comes easy. I shook hands with Admiral Byrd that evening and received his autographed book *Alone*, which sits in our library today. Admiral Byrd made five expeditions to Antarctica and was my childhood hero. I always intended to go there someday and, during my wait, I've lived vicariously through trips of others, including George and Trudy Huebner, who traveled there just a few years ago. You may recall that George was the head of the Redstone Missile Project for Chrysler Corporation and Trudy was the second woman to sit as a regent of our University. They were both in their 8th decade of life during this trip. Age was no boundary for new experiences for them.

All of us have boundaries defined or not, in our families; let me tell you of mine. I married my college sweetheart and for 44 years she has protected me from myself. That is no small feat. At the same time she guided our three children, Tim, Jeff, and Sarah, from being youngsters to becoming wonderful young adults. With their spouses they've all pushed boundaries. Let me brag a little bit about them.

Tim married Stacy and the two of them are well educated. Tim has two degrees from Stanford and a Michigan law degree, although his last year was spent at Harvard Law. He then entered a PhD degree program back at Stanford. Stacy has an undergraduated degree from Stanford and a law degree from Harvard. Our educational investment in Tim was a good investment. Nine years ago he and Stacy founded FindLaw, the most widely used law portal on the Internet. Stacy was the President and Tim was the Board Chair and CEO. Two years ago they sold it for more than my wife thinks it is polite to mention in public. Suffice it to say that they did very well and now have a second company.

Our second child, Jeff, is an otolaryngologist married to Kate, who is a pediatric neonatal intensivist. They now live in Fargo and both practice in a hospital nearly as large as ours. Jeff was made chief of the otolaryngology department 13 days ago, although I personally think he is too young to have such responsibility given his appearance clearly looking like a youngster, likely a result of his my wife's genes.

Our third child, Sarah, is a speech pathologist married to Ray, who is a geophysicist on the faculty at the University of Florida. They extended the boundary of our family with our first grandchild, Annie, and live in a home that is culturally rich, with Ray having been deeply involved with literature and the arts with a CD collection of more than 3,500 classical music discs.

My kids all believed in competition and all were varsity athletes at Huron High School here in Ann Arbor. Using running as the metaphor and yourself as the boundary they pushed the boundary of comfort and within themselves and developed a real sense of self-confidence not by beating someone else but being their own best. They ran marathons. Tim was our first nearly two decades ago. Sarah was the second, finishing three Boston's, and she was the fastest of our three children having come in 40th in Detroit to qualify for the Boston race. Kate and Jeff ran together in the Marine Corps Marathon and also in the Boston Marathon four years ago.

There is a lure about Boston and much of it is owed to Bill Rogers, who has spent time with my children. He is an Olympian and one who has run so many Bostons that his name is often synonymous with the run. The lure is also contagious, and I, too, at my daughter's behest, got off the couch and ran the 100th Boston marathon. Sarah then got me a poster autographed by Bill Rogers with a wonderful caption: "The race is not always for the swift but for those that keep on running." This is just as true in life. Many boundaries melt away with persistence.

As to myself I had many early boundaries. I grew up in East Lansing in a high school where the good times of "happy days" disappeared with football. That is where discipline hit the road. The boundaries were delivered by my coach, Vince Carillot, who had three rules (1) Winner's don't quit, Quitters don't win; (2) Sweat, Sacrifice, and a Little Extra Effort; and (3) Be a Gentlemen on and off the Field. There were no shortcuts. Many of my own students have heard modifications of these boundaries repeated as recently as last week.

I entered the University of Michigan as an engineering student and was deeply influenced by Thomas Dooley a missionary doctor, who provided care to the underserved in southeast Asia. He was the author of four books, which I read after my freshman year in engineering school, including *Before I Sleep*. He had many boundaries beyond himself. He established Medico and Project Care. The sick in his world were like a sad scene from "Live Aid." It had a profound effect on me and validated my perception of the physicians' social contract with humankind. I liked it! So I switched and became a premed student.

As I finished my four years in medical school I became accepted into the University's internal medicine residency, but Marion (Bill) DeWeese, with whom I spent six weeks as a senior extern, helped me cross another boundary. I decided to become a surgeon. Bill DeWeese was a remarkable gentleman and surgeon. He did the first aortorenal bypass, the first CABG in an animal, and created the first vena cava sieve to prevent fatal pulmonary embolism. His grace was profound. It's not only what you do but it is the way you do it, and he got it right.

My surgical training was interrupted by two years in the Army. I wore khaki greens not green scrubs as a General Medical Officer. I never saw Nam, but I served on the staff of a resolute officer who had an illustrative military career. Major General William Harris was a terror, in the mode of Patton. He had led the longest sustained drive in US Military history, over 120 miles in 24 hours representing the lower arm of the Inchon invasion that ended the Korean conflict. He was best known by his saying that "No one individual is more than important than the Corps." He was right. He was also a proud man. His hawkiness did not transform me but his pride did. Every single day with no exceptions in the nearly 40 years my family has lived in Ann Arbor we have displayed the American flag in front of our home: to say we are proud Americans is an understatement.

The boundaries of my residency were clearly defined by five individuals: Gardner Child, Jimmy Crudup, Jerry Turcotte, Bill Fry, and Cal Ernst.

Gardner Child was the Department of Surgery chair. I had 11 months on his service, more than any resident before or after, and his borders were very visible. He would frequently scold a trainee in the operating room" "Doctor, stop, think: how can you help me, not hinder me?" I never got this admonition but let me tell you I did think and think. Dr. Child hired me and gave me my first real job. Following his advice made sense.

Jimmy Crudup was an unusually gifted person. Jimmy became a technician working in the Department's surgical laboratories, after he lost his job in the labor-force during a wildcat strike in Detroit. He became absolutely outstanding in the research lab. He was as skilled a surgical technician as anyone that I have ever known. He could keep you out of trouble and had knowledge way beyond the classroom. I was actually quoted in newspapers out of state in a feature article written about him: "When Jimmy Crudup says, 'Doctor I was thinking' everyone stops and listens." It was sort of like "EF Hutton is my broker." Jimmy had grown up in the Deep South as an African American and taught me that the boundaries you are born with or raised with are not fixed. He was a real success.

Jerry Turcotte, who succeeded Dr. Child as chair, always said care for the patient, write about the disease. My first foray into writing about disease was what I consider boundary one, and that was to characterize renal artery fibrodysplasia. We succeeded with more than 100 contributions in the literature on this topic, including some sentinel work published nearly 25 years ago—with clarity, if I do say so myself—that has stood the test of time.

Bill Fry who was the first Coller professor and my mentor set the stage for the operative work with renal artery disease supported by the energy of Calvin Ernst, a longtime friend, with whom I later edited four textbooks.

All of this work was modified with some wonderful advice from Ralph Straffon, who had been the Chief of Surgery and CEO of the Cleveland Clinic. Ralph was a real Michigan man. He had been quarterback of the 1950 Michigan football team, a medical student here and a urology resident at the University. He was one of our most prominent alumni. His knowledge of renovascular hypertension provided stability to much of my early writings.

The second boundary was to search for an antithrombotic vascular graft using endothelial cells seeding as the method. We not only published nearly 40 articles on the subject but had continuous NIH funding for nearly two decades. The vast majority of this work was completed under the leadership of Linda Graham, a resident when she first took part in the research laboratory and later when she joined our faculty. Linda's talent as a clinician-scientist is unquestioned. She became the first woman to hold the presidency of the Society of University Surgeons and continues her research on vascular prostheses at the Cleveland Clinic Research Institute. She is a gem.

The third boundary related to the toxicity of protamine, a 21+ positive charged molecule, used clinically to reverse heparin anticoagulation. Tom Wakefield, working as resident in our laboratory, took the lead on this effort and with Phil Andrews, who was in charge of our protein sequencing laboratory at the University, allowed us to unmask some of the complications associated with this agent, including designing a protamine-like molecule with less toxicity, of which we own a patent.

The fourth boundary related to gene therapy. I doubt that one should ever seriously think about playing God, but an earlier cartoon in *Science* (when they actually had cartoons in their journal) depicted a very senior physician making rounds. He became disturbed by the younger people about him who only talked about making money, when in his earlier days playing God was enough of a reason to become a doctor. Such is foolishness but it does relate to the physician's responsibility of improving the human condition.

In the mid-1980s Michigan was in the vanguard of the evolving field of gene therapy, and vascular surgery was responsible for one of four groups comprising Bill Kelly's gene therapy program. All of this started with a hallmark paper in *Science* in 1989 with Betsy Nabel as the senior author. No p values, but an exceedingly important novel observation that a new gene in transplanted cells could produce a new protein in a living animal. That was a first. Betsy was also an intellectual leader and after her career at Michigan she became Head of the Heart and Lung and Blood Institute at the National Institutes of Health. She too is a gem.

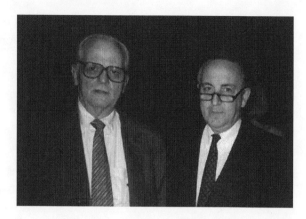

The author and
Stanley Crawford

As a more senior faculty member, many boundaries have become clear, set by others who have all been major players. Let me speak first about the men: Lazar Greenfield, George Zuidema, Gil Omenn, Stanley Crawford, Jack Jacobson, and Mike Mulholland.

Lazar Greenfield and his caval filter have saved thousands of lives. He also with the stroke of a pen created the Section of Vascular Surgery at the medical school, an action that I am very thankful for. A number of years ago the medical school hosted its 150th anniversary and invited all of the past deans and vice presidents, following which a program occurred at Hill Auditorium. Included were the vice presidents, the first of which was George Zuidema, who gave me a key to the surgical OR lab when I was a junior medical student before he became the Chair of Surgery at Johns Hopkins; and Gil Omenn, who facilitated the Cardio-vascular Center project. Without Gil it would likely still have been an architect's drawing. Mike Mulholland, my current chair, is a committed scientist. He is more willing to take a risk to make a better scientific institution than anyone I know.

Stanley Crawford is the most endearing of contemporary vascular surgeons and he changed my view of boundary risk. He took on the sickest and pushed the technical envelope. He treated thoracoabdomi-nal aneurysms like no one else had, and today we all do as he did. We are indebted to him.

And then there is Jack Jacobson. He became an umpteen millionaire by developing microvascular surgical instruments. He is a cultured New Yorker who actually had his early education at the University of Toledo.

I have the upmost respect for him. He is a major philanthropist who created the American College of Surgeons Jacobson Award, a number of NIH programs, and has espoused a sense of philanthropy of giving back to his community which I embrace with my entire being.

In 2003, Jack Jacobson published a book entitled *The Classical Music Experience,* which included two CDs narrated by his neighbor Kevin Kline. I have given this book to many of my colleagues attempting to tramp out country music and to improve the culture, but honestly it is an experiment—country music dies hard in the operating room. Music has opened many boundaries for me. I've always thought of the big "three" in Southeast Michigan not referring to the automotive industry, but being U of M athletics, the Medical Center, and the University Music Society. I still think I've got it right.

There are a number of other boundary setters within the gentler gender. They have restructured boundaries far more than I would admit. These boundary makers include my wife, Nancy, and daughter, Sarah; Caroline Jobst; my nurses, Charleen Minard, Elaine Fellows, and Becky Bertha; and my secretary, Duwana Villemure.

Nancy has been my sonar piece as I approached many boundaries and Sarah, my daughter, has given me the charge to "Go for it." When you are in your 6th decade of life and have never run a marathon that is some "going".

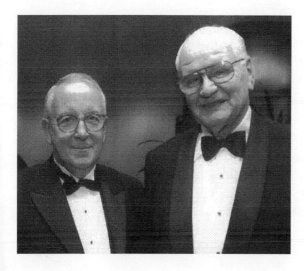

The author and
Julius (Jack)
Jacobson

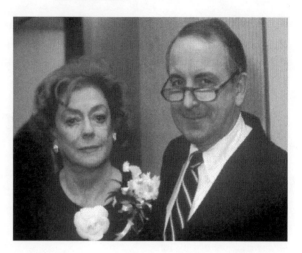

Caroline Jobst and
the author

Then there is Caroline Jobst, whose 4-million-dollar gift established our research laboratories. She broke down many walls and boundaries for women in business, and she endowed the things that will continue to break down many boundaries of ignorance as our laboratory is successful in its research endeavors.

And there are our nurses. The three, Charlene Minard, Elaine Fellows, and Becky Bertha, have been in the clinic, in the operating rooms, the emergency room. They are absolutely fantastic at helping patients cross many different boundaries, and they deserve to have statues built for them.

And, of course there is my secretary, Duwana Villemure. She has been my office confident and organizer for nearly 2 ½ decades. She is professional, efficient, and loyal. She also knows more about me and my shortcomings than I want anyone else to know. I treat her with great respect and she deserves it—and I'm very beholden to her.

And there are today's leaders of the Cardiovascular Center: Linda Larin, Kim Eagle, Rich Prager, and David Pinsky. They are pushing a real boundary against the number one killer in our country and they are all for real. Kim is a superb cardiologist and demographer; Rich Prager is the surgeons' surgeon who I would want to fix my heart should the need arise; and David Pinsky who is a scholarly intellect and mature scientist.

I and the other three CVC medical directors are blessed with the presence of Linda Larin, who has been glue of the Center's birthing and evolution. From my perspective she has been one of the most resolute administrative leaders in our Institution during my entire career at the health system.

I've had many faculty partners and vascular fellows who have trained with us. Most importantly, the trainees have probably educated the faculty and me as much as we have trained them.

Then there is David Handleman, my benefactor. David is a rare human being. He is someone we should wish were part of our family. David is smart, humble, nice, and very generous. I can't thank him enough for the Professorship that carries his name. It provides a symbol of integrity at improving the care of patients.

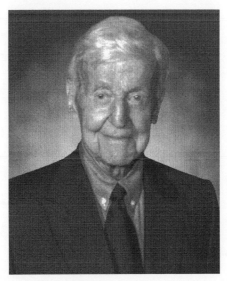

David Handleman

Use your imagination—just think how lucky I've been for nearly a half century to learn at and serve the University of Michigan. Lastly, to paraphrase a recent sentiment, let me remind you of what you have seen today: it's about working together as a team to get beyond the boundaries, and that's the Michigan difference.

Godspeed to all.

18

A LIFE'S PERSPECTIVE:

THE STANLEY PROFESSORSHIP

This address was read by the author as part of the University of Michigan inauguration of the James C. Stanley Professorship in Vascular Surgery on July 27, 2012, in Ann Arbor. Thomas W. Wakefield was the honored recipient of the Professorship.

It's a rare occasion for me to be addressing a few hundred of my colleagues and friends on a topic unrelated to science, and it's an even rarer opportunity for me to try to sum up the essence of my life, while acknowledging those who've made my journey so memorable.

My parents, both born in 1900, had seen my brother, Bob, grow through childhood, when I arrived in 1938. They gave me a lot of freedom as I stumbled through adolescence in another college town, East Lansing, during the "happy days" in the middle of the last century. It was a different era. Life was peaceful. You didn't lock your front door at night or your car at work, and life seemed easy. Getting 100% on an exam was not so hard and classroom discipline was never an issue.

On the athletic field that wasn't always so. My football coach, Vince Carillot, expected 110% of us, and discipline was palpable. It was there I learned to get beyond myself during the two years I played varsity ball for him; it wasn't about me, it was about the game. It was about competing and we did well—ranked #1 in the state my senior year until we lost to Battle Creek Lakeview in the season's final game. I am sure that neither the coach nor I will forget that loss and therein was a lesson: losing is detestable. Coach Carillot figured it out, made the right changes, and his team went undefeated the next year, but it was too late for those of us who were seniors. I haven't forgotten—and in the clinical arena a

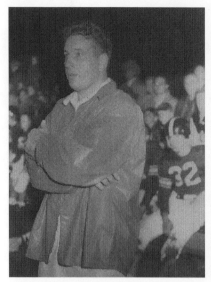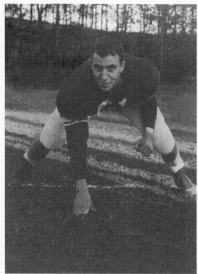

Coach Vince Carillot and the author, 1955

half-century later I have never been willing to accept an irretrievable loss on behalf of my patients, for it to be too late for them. It started with football, and some may have thought it was only about winning in those days, but most of us knew it was about never losing.

Vince was different; he had played football at Michigan State, was our high school coach, became head backfield coach at State, then head coach at Tulsa, and then—get this—left coaching, came to the University of Michigan, and received his PhD in the economics of higher education before becoming the vice president of Eastern Michigan University. Was he competitive? Of course. If any of you think I might be too competitive, I'm happy to acknowledge that I first acquired that trait when I played for him. My coach, Vince Carillot, is here today from Georgia, to help me celebrate this event.

It was 1956 when I first left home and traveled to Ann Arbor to enter the university as a student in the College of Engineering. I began medical school four years later. The medical campus didn't look the same in 1960; it was much simpler. And it was in Ann Arbor that I met and fell in love with my wife of 50 years, Nancy. We met as young undergraduate students, and her dark eyes and gentle ways made courting her easy. We were married shortly after I finished my first year in medical school. We had started our life together.

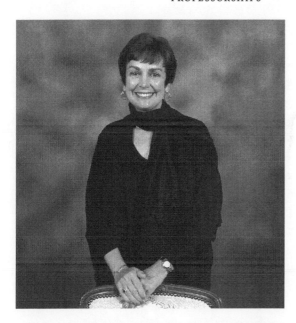

My wife, Nancy

Three years after being married, as I began my internship, our first child, Tim, arrived, followed a few years later by Jeff and then Sarah. As youngsters these three were the apples of their mother's and my eyes, and they have remained so as adults. Joy has no equal when your children are successful and healthy. Each have married and I'm proud of their—

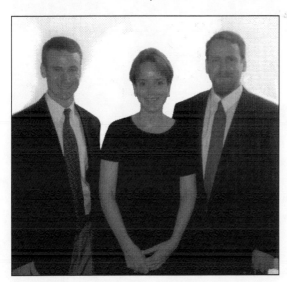

Our children: Jeffrey, Sarah, Timothy

and their spouses'—choices: to make a difference in others' lives. All six have careers serving others in education, law, or medicine. We couldn't have wished more of them. We have four grandchildren—pure glee—and all heart and lungs with energy to spare. Life has been good to us. So be it for them.

Make no mistake about it: the centerfold of the Stanley family was and is Nancy. She's been my comforter, my confessor, and my companion without whom I never would have found contentment and happiness among the rigors of life. She was always there at day's end and was the reason I would awake every morning with an awareness of what a wonderful world it is.

I had some real heroes in medical school and during my residency. The Medical faculty was very small in those days compared to today, but our teachers were extraordinary. I had been accepted into the Internal Medicine residency when my career changed course and I followed the advice of Dr. Marion (Bill) DeWeese, on whose surgical service I had rotated as a senior, and who had performed the world's first bypass to a kidney. I entered the surgery residency.

Two other individuals had a major impact on my learning during my residency: The first was Cal Ernst, who taught me the value of hard work and how to write. He invested well; we later shared the editorship of the *Journal of Vascular Surgery*, our specialty's most widely read journal. The second was the Departmental Chair, Gardner Child. I spent 11 months with him in the operating theater during my four years of training. He was an eloquent surgeon whose deceptive technical expertise made the most difficult procedure look simple. I truly wanted to be like him. Most importantly Dr. Child underwrote my appointment as an NIH Trainee in Academic Surgery and that was the spark during my residency that introduced me to bench research.

Any successes that evolved from my early days in the lab were clearly eclipsed by a remarkable gift in 1987 from Carolyn Jobst, who funded our research laboratories in honor of her late husband, Conrad. Those were heady days. It was more about dis-

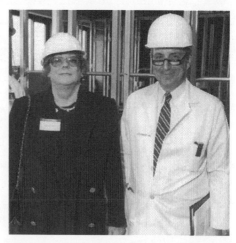

Caroline Jobst and the author, at the construction site of the Conrad Jobst Research Laboratories

covery than worrying about grants and the indirect dollars they might generate. Among the many investigations we pursued, I remain particularly proud of three.

The first involved a 35-year sojourn on the study of arterial fibrodysplasia. One result of our efforts is that the University has since become a destination for those afflicted with this disease. Nearly a hundred reports have emanated from this work, of which many remain benchmark contributions.

The second occurred when I was a young staff member working with Bill Burkel in the Anatomy-Cell Biology Department, and mentoring a resident, Linda Graham. Our laboratory at that time had a focus on seeding endothelium on vascular grafts. This effort was NIH-funded for many years. That funding has continued uninterrupted in Linda's lab at the Cleveland Clinic Research Institute today. Linda is a superb vascular surgeon and outstanding scientist. A few years after she planted her roots in our laboratories she became the first woman to be President of the Society of University Surgeons.

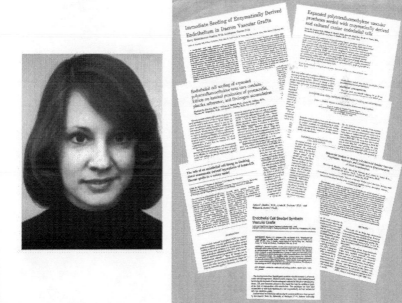

Linda Graham and endothelial cell seeding of vascular grafts

The third work occurred when as a more senior faculty member I had the good fortune to be involved with some of the country's early gene transfer studies, working with two new faculty members, Betsy Nabel and her husband, Gary. This work resulted in many publications, led by her seminal paper in *Science* in 1989, the first to document the expression of a gene in cells transplanted into a living subject. Betsy recently assumed the presidency of Brigham and Women's Hospital in Boston after being the Director of the Heart, Lung and Blood Institute of the NIH, and I am delighted that she is here today to share in this celebration.

I was 17 when I first came to Ann Arbor, and my age had doubled, when at 34 I joined the faculty in 1972. I'm exceedingly grateful to the many who have helped me since those early days, especially the trainees from whom I've learned as much as I've given them, and to the faculty partners who have kept me on track. My clinical and academic life also has been particularly blessed by three exceptional nurses: Charleen Minard, Elaine Fellows, and Becky Bertha; and especially by Duwana

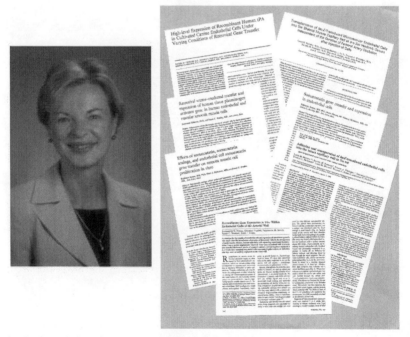

Elizabeth Nabel and gene transfer into endothelial cells

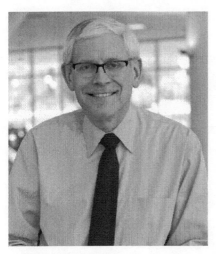

Thomas Wakefield

Villemure, my secretary of more than 30 years. She has made my sailing smooth during more turbulent days than I can count. I am very, very grateful to her.

I had nearly doubled my age again, when at 66 Tom Wakefield assumed the office I had occupied for nearly 30 years, the Head of the Section of Vascular Surgery. What a win for our specialty at Michigan. Tom's a great clinician and scientist. He and I have coauthored 71 papers and 17 chapters, and hold a number of patents from our laboratory efforts. The formal written conclusion of the search committee seeking my successor was that Dr. Wakefield was their number 1, 2, and 3 choice. Not bad considering that the other candidates, all excellent academics, were from Harvard, Washington University, and Stanford. I was very proud of Tom then as I am today.

The Medical Campus in 2012 has changed dramatically since my days as an M-1. It's become a beacon for care, education, and scientific discovery. My personal good fortune took a big leap when David Handleman endowed a professorship, which to this day I hold. David's first wife had been a patient of mine. He oversaw what was arguably the world's most successful CD recording company. Therein was an additional bond I shared with him—music. Music has a special place in my existence, be it in the operating room or at a University Musical Society (UMS) performance at Hill Auditorium. It's more than a simple connection. To me it's the rhythm of life.

I've been privileged to meet many in the arts, like Yo-Yo Ma, Wynton Marsalis, and Valery Gergiev from St Petersburg, Russia, one of the world's most eminent conductors. I'm a little bit of a groupie. Talking to or sharing a meal with these icons has been a dream come true for me, with the clear hope that my linear life might be bettered if just a little of their artistry and creativity would rub off. Only in Ann Arbor with our treasured UMS could a busy surgeon have such a treat.

If enjoying a rich professional life wasn't enough, five years ago we opened up the University's Cardiovascular Center—a showplace and place of extraordinary care. All of the directors took part in the dedication, but I think I had the best part—introducing both our University President, Mary Sue Coleman, and someone I mentored as a medical student and young surgical resident, the keynote speaker, Sanjay Gupta. The Cardiovascular Center has a unique group of Directors who have by all accounts brought significant credit to the University Hospital and Medical School—with an acknowledgment by all four of us who are physicians that Linda Larin, with her administrative and people skills, has been the glue behind the Center's success.

There is a third group, beyond my family and colleagues, to whom I am very grateful. They are the many patients I've operated upon during the past four decades. They entrusted me with their lives and have revealed to me the best of the human spirit. Let me share two patient stories, in hopes that you will understand a little more of my life as a vascular surgeon.

The first is about Jake Zangara, a poster child for our center if ever there was one, who had severe hypertension from both renal arteries being obstructed. He was only three months old, weighed only 11

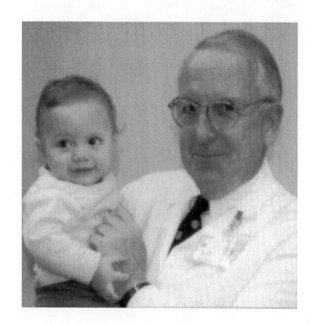

The author and Jake Zangara, the youngest child to undergo a renal artery reconstruction.

pounds, and had two cardiac arrests in New York City before being flown to Ann Arbor in 2006 for emergency surgery to reconstruct his renal arteries. It worked, and after waiting for the eight hours we spent in the operating room, his parents, both physicians from the East Coast, could finally share a sigh of relief. He's now a bright young six-year-old living with his sister and younger brother. His parents are here today to help celebrate the inauguration of this professorship.

The second story is about Sam Eldersveld, who had been Chair of the University's Political Science Department in the late 1960s; had been our city's mayor; and on a Tuesday morning in 2005 ruptured an aortic aneurysm. He was 87 years old and the survival for a free rupture at that age is less than 10%. He was rushed from the ER to the OR for emergent surgery and we helped him beat the odds. Three years later Sam published his 23rd book at age 90. I had an unusual relationship with him. You see, in 1959 when he was on a sabbatical, four of us had rented his home to live in during our senior year as undergraduates. He was a world-class academic who taught at the University for 54 years—and how lucky I was to have been able to help him see the end of the day that Tuesday. Sam's wife is here with us today.

Both these patients, nine decades apart in age, are what my practice had morphed into. As a surgeon in many difficult circumstances you know the statistics may be against you, but you have to be resolute to take on the challenge—patients and their families expect and deserve that. This is not always a simple undertaking. The fact is that there is no room to start over once the operation has started, and you have to finish. It's about going the extra yard and finishing every time we go to the operating room. There's no alternative. It's not the macho lifestyle of surgeons portrayed in the media or the hospital margin that counts. If you're a clinician the only thing that counts at the end of the day is the wellness of your patient.

It may sound like I always knew where I was going, but I didn't. Life and the universe are too complex to be that factual, but I always knew who I was. I was not ambitious but I did carry expectations for myself. Some were pretty ethereal, but I believe they enabled my life to have meaning. As a teacher I've never been hesitant to share them many times with youth who have come my way, so let me repeat them to the young in this hall today.

Reject mediocrity. The unimportance of being average is staggering. Just getting by in life doesn't make sense. I view the wasting of one's potential as a perennial scourge. You don't have to be the best at anything, but don't settle for being average at everything. Find your niche and go at it.

Be creative. Leave something behind you that will outlive you—a story, a painting, a song, an idea. Something of your own doing, not bought or borrowed from another, something for future generations. Lasting creativity with your hands, voice, and mind is a blessing we don't share with lesser life on this planet. It's a human gift—don't waste it.

Do not be risk adverse. Don't hesitate to venture beyond boundaries that are likely to disclose new wonders, especially those that awaken your mind. After all, discovery usually is much more likely to occur beyond known and safe horizons. For those of you who want to make a difference taking risks should be part of your mantra.

Be tolerant. Embrace the colors and sounds of human diversity for they are the essence of life. Your journey will be brighter for the experience and the world will make more sense along the way. And keep your moral compass in plain sight. I admonish you to abhor anyone carrying an ill-founded bias against another human being.

Don't be silent. I've seen the damning effects of silence. I have witnessed the unwillingness of some to see the loss of dignity and purpose in individuals they are at ease in ignoring. It's painful to observe them, and I often find myself struggling to call them out. I don't believe in remaining silent. A certain degree of personal integrity exists in speaking up at a moment that is more important than you are. There are always excuses to being silent. Don't accept them.

Be patient with those about you. The fact is that the slow and less well-informed will always outnumber you. Many will be loud and callous and you can't avoid them, try as you may. My advice: be patient, for at day's end the loud will be silent, and perhaps the next morning's light will find them in a different place.

Be content with yourself. Seek peace within your own daily existence. It may come from your faith or a simple appreciation of life's complexities arising from our DNA beginnings. You needn't feign away from your beliefs; in fact, your beliefs will shape your life as much as your life's circumstances will mold your beliefs.

Share yourself with others without conditions or design. You will receive much more in return without asking. Avoid being insular and accept human contact, even when you are vulnerable. More than anything else sharing of self will give your life balance.

When I was a little boy, growing up in another college town, we had neighbors on either side of our home who were university professors, and I think I often dreamed of growing up so I too could be called a "learned" person. I wanted to do something real, and, of course, I wanted my life to make a difference. My path has been blessed with many riches, given to me from the university, from my colleagues and trainees, my patients, and my family, especially my wife, Nancy. So here I am, seven decades later, and it all has happened. I am very lucky. And so are all of us within the shadows of our University, which created today a Professorship in my family's name. Many, many thanks.

Peace to you all.

CHALLENGES

Offering advice to the young is often fraught with the risk of being considered arrogant or, worse yet, being ignored altogether. These two addresses are my challenges and recommendations first to a few hundred young surgeons in Scotland as they near completion of their surgical training, and second to a wide array of more than 1,500 students in the United States who are about to enter the larger world, having just received their university's undergraduate and graduate degrees. The young of both groups are special, and speaking to them allowed me to bare my own wishes for a betterment of humankind. They are our future. As I addressed them I was most cognizant of their value to both me and society.

19

ON BEING A SURGEON AND
THE HUMAN CONDITION

This brief address was read before the Royal College of Surgeons, Edinburgh, at their Annual Fellowship Convocation on June 12, 1992, in Edinburgh, Scotland. The author was the recipient of an Honorary Fellowship. on that occasion.

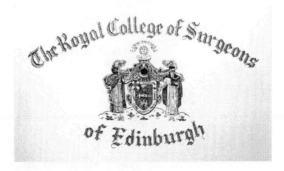

I wish to extend my deepest gratitude to the Royal College for my honorary fellowship—no greater recognition can one receive from one's peers. My comments today are addressed to the new fellows on being a surgeon and the human condition: where you as a person fit, and where your profession fits. At times there will seem to be precious little room for both. My comments are personal, not the terse facts usually attributed to a scientist, editor, or professor. They are meant to reveal a side of me, and perhaps of yourselves, that others rarely see, but perhaps should.

Fellowship in this College is recognition of intellectual accomplishments and technical mastery in the craft of surgery. These are not trivial or simple givens, but as you know, perhaps more than your mentors and teachers know, these achievements came about as the result of consider-able sacrifice, and extra effort. But what does this mean to you tomorrow or a quarter of a century from now when you find yourself in my shoes, as a more senior surgeon, wondering what your efforts have meant?

I would hope your Fellowship will give you the opportunity to learn more of yourself and mankind than might otherwise be the case. Given all the insight of training, of walking on the very edge of life and death with your patients in the operating theatre, of the recognition of the finiteness of life, and the examinations—given all of this, certainly, judg-ments and action have been engrained in your everyday lives. You must learn to use these tools wisely.

There is a verse entitled Desiderata, inscribed on the wall of an old Baltimore church in my country, that bears witness to yourselves. Let me share its contents with you. I hope you find a bit of yourself in its words.

Go placidly among the noise and haste,
and remember what peace there may be in silence.
As far as possible without surrender
be on good terms with all persons.

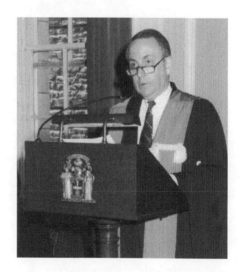

The author at the podium
addressing the initiates of the
Royal College of Surgeons,
Edinburgh

Speak your truth quietly and clearly;
and listen to others,
even the dull and the ignorant;
they too have their story.

Avoid loud and aggressive persons,
they are vexations to the spirit.
If you compare yourself with others,
you may become vain and bitter,
for always there will be greater and lesser persons than yourself.

Enjoy your achievements as well as your plans.

Keep interested in your own career, however humble;
it is a real possession in the changing fortunes of time.
Exercise caution in your business affairs;
for the world is full of trickery.

But let this not blind you to what virtue there is;
many persons strive for high ideals;
and everywhere life is full of heroism.

Be yourself.
Especially, do not feign affection.
Neither be cynical about love;
for in the face of all aridity and disenchantment
it is as perennial as the grass.

Take kindly the counsel of the years,
gracefully surrendering the things of youth.

Nurture strength of spirit to shield you in sudden misfortune.
But do not distress yourself with dark imaginings.
Many fears are born of fatigue and loneliness,
Beyond a wholesome discipline,
be gentle with yourself.

You are a child of the universe,
no less than the trees and the stars;
you have a right to be here.

And whether or not it is clear to you,
no doubt the universe is unfolding as it should.
Therefore be at peace with God,
whatever you conceive him to be.

And whatever your labors and aspirations,
in the noisy confusion of life keep peace with your soul.

With all its sham, drudgery, and broken dreams,
it is still a beautiful world.
Be cheerful.
Strive to be happy.

These words by Max Ehrmann are as poignant to us today as when they were written more than 65 years ago. "Be cheerful. Strive to be happy." For those of us given the opportunity to help our fellow beings that's certainly doable.

I'm a very fortunate surgeon. My work has given me great joy. Caring for the sick has no equal. Your vantage point is unique—to see, hands on, the problems of society in the needs for shelter, for food, for companionship, and to recognize the importance of family for sustenance of spirit as well as body. Being a surgeon is a hard-earned privilege, but it should bring one great satisfaction.

Like you, I live in a free society with great abundance and I've been blessed in loving and having been loved by friends and family, including my wife, Nancy, who is here with us in this hall today. I would like to offer you a simple observation paraphrased from an early American writer, Ralph Waldo Emerson, one that has influenced most of my own personal actions and professional life. Simply put it is that:

"The best purpose in life is to use it for something that will outlive it."

In receiving the Fellowship in the College, you have been given a gift. Use it wisely. If you do, there will be no difficulty in sorting out where you and your profession fit into the human condition. If you give something back to mankind that will outlive yourself, you will surely find happiness.

This is a special day for you who have received your diplomas. To the new fellows, my congratulations and best wishes for the future wisdom and good that will come to you. Be proud of your accomplishments. Enjoy the community of surgeons throughout our ever-shrinking globe…remember we are all children of the same universe.

Godspeed.

20

RELEVANCE AND RESPONSIBILITY

*This Commencement Address was delivered to the undergraduate, gradu-
ate students, teachers, staff, executive officers, and governing Board members of the University of Toledo on December 18, 2010, in Toledo, Ohio. The
author was the recipient of an Honorary Doctor of Science Degree on that
occasion.*

My congratulations to each and every one of you on this day of your
graduation—on your being among a select few of humankind to have
even ever had the opportunity to learn of the world and yourselves by
attending a university.

For just one moment think about the others on this globe who have
not been as fortunate as you. Realize how special your journey has been.
And be aware that the opportunities that will unfold in your future will
outnumber by far those of preceding generations, including those of
mine and your teachers at the University of Toledo.

After today your paths are likely to be quite diverse. That's a given.
But tomorrow two questions will begin surfacing for all of you: First,
what's the real value of your education? And second, will you use your
newfound knowledge meaningfully?

The answer depends on your inner self. That's where your core values
reside. It's your relevant side, and your outer self. That's what you do.
That's what others see. It's your responsible side.

Two simple concepts: what your inner self is, and what your outer
self does.

Let's talk about you. For years many of you've had family, friends, and
teachers lead and push you to succeed. They set boundaries from your
childhood to today. Most were protective. They kept you on time, kept

you healthy, and many kept you safe. Almost all were focused inward, centered on you and your behavior.

In contrast, the most important boundaries you will face after today will beg you to look outward. They are not about you. They are where tomorrow's frontiers exist. And they are likely to be a long way from the security of those that have supported you in the past.

Many of these boundaries will be beyond your comfort zone, but you will be the better for finding and exploring them. Getting beyond those boundaries is where you will grow. It's where discovery occurs of both yourself and the world.

It is there that you will find the new, expected or not. Such may take a toll on your emotional and physical energy, but, clearly, getting across these boundaries will be less burdensome if you know where you came from and where you're going. It is, then, that what you have learned and know becomes singularly important. And that's what your education has been all about. That's no surprise, especially today.

As you approach certain boundaries you may find yourself on your own with choices—and you must choose wisely. My advice, just for a moment, is to stop listening to those who helped you get to today and listen to yourself. Some of you have been pursuing the goals of others for years, and you've been making choices not always of your own making. It may have gotten you this far, but pleasing others at the expense of being relevant to your own self carries risks. You need to claim your own inner self. Sort out the real and imagined future you desire. It belongs to no one else.

So on a heady day like today, take time to decide who you are and what you really believe in. Simply define your own values. And don't forget to be honest with yourself and authentic to others. Clearly, having an uncertain persona is better than a false one. And remember, having a persona thrust on you by others will not last, for soon they will not be there. You and you alone will determine your inner self, your core values.

You have been well-prepared for this by your teachers at the University of Toledo. They have tried to connect you to the real world. And for the most part they've succeeded. Your diploma speaks to that. But tomorrow they will no longer serve as your intermediaries and you will find yourself alone with the joys and sufferings of the world.

On good days you may have a litany of opportunities, too many to take on—all at once. And you'll wish your teachers were at your side to help you make the right choice. On other days the issues may not be of your making, but they may affect you nevertheless. Some will be daunting: hunger, illiteracy, illness, poverty, unsustainable consumption of precious goods, societal violence, and on and on and on. There are no guarantees that your path will be easy.

As you mend your way, the technology and industry of your generation will provide many tools that can make a difference—tools unavailable to earlier generations. But use them wisely. In that regard, I fervently hope you will be contributors to a better world, not simply be consumers of our earth's shrinking resources. I believe how you confront the problems and opportunities of the next half-century will spell out your success and will define the future of your community.

There will be many changes. And you will experience them for better or worse. You may object to some changes, but don't waste too much time objecting. You're better off finding those that fit your inner and outer self—and then spend your energies embracing them.

With the right choices you will transform yourself and you will likely transform the community in which you reside. At times it may be difficult—economic challenges, political battles, unresponsive people to help you. So be it. But your share of the difficulties will not be so heavy if you possess the agility and imagination that has seen you to this day. In fact, the breadth of the education you have received at the University will serve you well in this regard.

I have deep roots in Ohio and Toledo. My father was born and grew up in Southern Ohio and my mother was born in Toledo and attended Scott High, just a few miles from campus. I love this community and have the greatest admiration for the faculty and staff who have guided you through the past few years. The University of Toledo is a gem of an institution of higher learning. Many of its noteworthy alumni and esteemed academic leaders are my dear friends.

In thinking of the circumstances of today, I seriously pondered what I might want to hear if I were in your seats. In my days, parents and teachers frequently said "get a job and work hard." If I were in your seats today, that would go in one ear and out the other—and it certainly wouldn't challenge me, at least not in a way I might wish.

Now remember, I told you how important I thought it was for you to define yourself, to separate yourself for a moment from the expectations of others. You know people like me, and listen to yourself. So, in some regards, I'm not too sure you should listen too intently to me. But you know I may be a little more objective than the others. After all until today I had no vested interest in placing my own thoughts on your table.

When I was your age I had many expectations for myself, and most have stuck with me through the years. Most were pretty ethereal, but I believe they enabled my life to have meaning. With a half-century of being married to my college sweetheart, three wonderful and productive children, more academic accolades than I deserved, and a lot of gratitude from those I've served—my own expectations may be of value on your table.

Let me paint a scenario of what I might ask of you before you reach my age. I want you to discover your place in the human condition. If you revel in the flatness of our world, create something on your own, learn to live with the difficult; and grow with others, then you will have found that place. None of this is too much to expect of university graduates, and it's not too much for me to ask of you. So here are my expectations. There are eight of them.

First, be adventurous. Don't hesitate to venture beyond boundaries that are likely to disclose new wonders, especially those that awaken your intellect and humanity. Somewhere along the way consider your role in serving and helping others. That's an important element of a learned society. And that is the society to which you have entered today with your graduation.

Second, be tolerant. Embrace the colors and sounds of human diversity for they are the essence of life. Your journey will be brighter for the experience and the world will make more sense along the way. And keep your moral compass in plain sight. I admonish you to abhor anyone carrying an ill-founded bias against another human being. Understanding the value that lies in differences among people across cultures and societies is requisite to building a better world. You need to be part of that and you will, but only if you allow yourself to see the true value of diversity.

Third, don't be silent. I've seen the damning effects of silence. I have witnessed the unwillingness of some to see the loss of dignity and purpose in individuals they are at ease in ignoring. It's painful to observe them, and I often find myself struggling to call them out. But I don't believe in remaining silent. A certain degree of personal integrity exists in speaking up at a moment that is more important than you are. There are always excuses to being silent. The point of your education is to give you the ability to speak clearly and be heard.

Fourth, reject mediocrity. The unimportance of being average is staggering. Just getting by in your life's work doesn't make sense and is not what your education has prepared you for. I view the wasting of one's potential as a perennial scourge. Unfortunately, not giving your all is commonplace and seems to be a ubiquitous contributor to mediocrity. Don't allow your inner or outer self to be part of this. You don't have to be the best at anything, but don't settle for being average.

Fifth, be patient with those about you. The fact is that the slow and less well-informed will always outnumber you. Many will be loud and callous and you can't avoid them, try as you may. My advice: be patient, for at day's end the loud will be silent, and perhaps the next morning's light will find them in a different place. And when you can, offer the slow and uninformed help to attain what you now have.

Sixth, be creative. Leave something behind you that will outlive you—a story, a painting, a song, an idea. Something of your own doing, not bought or borrowed from another, something for future generations. Lasting creativity with your hands, voice, and mind is a blessing we don't share with lesser life on this planet. It's a human gift. And don't stifle creativity, it's too valuable to defer to one's waning days. Waiting may come too late.

Seventh: find contentment. Seek peace within your daily existence. It may come from your faith or a simple appreciation of life's complexities, from our DNA beginnings to our cultural breadth. You needn't feign away from your beliefs. In fact, your beliefs will shape your life as much as your life's circumstances will mold your beliefs. Whichever it is, I hope it will bring contentment within the chaos of life.

Eighth, and last, seek happiness. Most importantly, share yourself with others without conditions or design. You will receive much more in return—without asking. Avoid being insular and accept human contact, even when you are vulnerable. Indeed, happiness born of friendship will enrich your life far more than all your other accomplishments.

Again, congratulations on your achievement today. I share in your pride.

And remember: keep your inner self relevant and your outer self responsible. It is my deepest hope that with those underpinnings you will continue to grow and better humankind.

Peace.

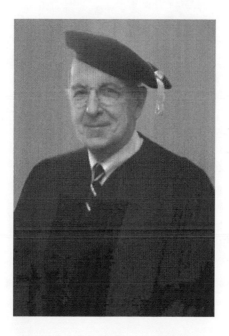

The author in academic regalia at the Commencement

ACKNOWLEDGEMENTS

The author is most appreciative of the copy editing by Marcia LaBrenz and the production efforts of Paula Newcomb. I am particularly grateful to H. Christopher Hedly of Michigan MultiMedia who developed the graphic contributions to this work. Very special recognition is given to my administrative assistant of nearly four decades, Duwana Villemure, who retrieved and formatted all of the book's presentations. Lastly, my deepest thanks to Nancy, my wife of more than five decades, who supported me through the many years these addresses were evolving.